100 mg
twice a day

The New Arthritis
Breakthrough

Also by Henry Scammell

SCLERODERMA:
The Proven Therapy That Can Save Your Life

The New Arthritis Breakthrough

Henry Scammell

M. EVANS

Lanham • New York • Boulder • Toronto • Plymouth, UK

Published by M. Evans
An imprint of The Rowman & Littlefield Publishing Group,
Inc.
4501 Forbes Boulevard, Suite 200, Lanham, Maryland 20706

Estover Road
Plymouth PL6 7PY
United Kingdom

Distributed by NATIONAL BOOK NETWORK

LCCN: 97-061592
ISBN-13: 978-0-87131-843-5
ISBN-10: 0-87131-843-1

In loving memory of
Thomas McPherson Brown,
Physician
1906–1989

ASK YOUR DOCTOR

This book does not substitute for the medical advice and supervision of your personal physician. No medical therapy should be undertaken except under the direction of a physician.

If it has been medically determined that you are suffering from a form of inflammatory arthritis, lupus, or scleroderma, your physician should have the opportunity to read this book, to learn about the infectious etiology of the disease and its treatment with the safe, clinically tested, and proven therapy that it describes.

Contents

Let's Start with the Proof

During the past several years, hundreds of newspaper and television reports on the successful use of antibiotic therapy for arthritis have repeatedly raised public expectation of a major shift in direction for the treatment of mankind's most widespread crippling disease. Until very recently, however, those expectations were routinely disappointed in the doctor's office where they were usually dismissed as premature, inconclusive, or, not infrequently, as quackery.

"THE DISEASE CAN BE SUPPRESSED . . ."

There are now signs that the old pattern of hope and denial is about to end. In mid-November of 1997, unprecedented levels of improvement and remission for arthritis patients treated with a safe, inexpensive antibiotic therapy were verified in a presentation to the American College of Rheumatology. At the ACR Annual Scientific Meeting in Washington, D.C., a Nebraska

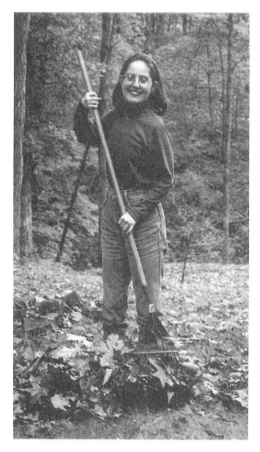

Lori Fillenwarth, Indianapolis, Ind., had RA for twenty-two years before learning of antibiotic therapy in 1995.

Up to then I'd been given all the usual toxic drugs. The gold injections caused oozing sores in my mouth and lips and a growth on my tongue; the methotrexate damaged my liver; the nitrogen mustard put me into menopause at age 27. Who knows what the cortisone, indocin, plaquenil, Imuran, azulfadine, clinoril, etc. did to me.

Despite the drugs, I steadily went downhill. Nausea kept my weight below 100 pounds. I had replacements of both shoulders, a hip and an elbow, couldn't wear regular shoes and felt pain in every joint. I used a three-wheel cart to get around my office and a wheelchair elsewhere. My husband carried me on the stairs and to the sofa or car, and often he had to bathe and dress me. My hands were claws that wouldn't close and I needed narcotics or muscle relaxers to sleep.

Then the miracle happened. I have been praying and taking minocycline since April 1995, reducing the oral cortisone and giving up all other medications. For the first time in twenty years I have no swelling in any joints and am not anemic. I no longer use the wheelchair and I'm no longer exhausted. I can cook, shop, clean house, rake leaves, climb stairs, and take walks with ease and without pain. I sleep well, eat like a horse, have gained five pounds, and am regaining some muscle tone. My doctor is amazed. Joe and I are overjoyed. It's like beginning a new, second life.

researcher named James O'Dell, M.D., described to some 4,000 physicians the results of a three-year follow-up study on a small group of patients who had responded positively to such therapy in the initial stages of their illness. "If rheumatoid arthritis is treated early and aggressively," his report concluded, "the disease can be suppressed, and patients will benefit. . . . [The antibiotic] minocycline may act on an infectious process or trigger . . . that is helping cause or perpetuate rheumatoid arthritis."

O'Dell had the numbers to prove it, and in short order this newest chapter in the story of a major arthritis breakthrough was sweeping the country.

But would it be believed? And would patients with inflammatory arthritis now be able to receive this therapy?

While Dr. O'Dell's announcement appeared to offer the best possible news to arthritis sufferers, it created serious political problems for the ACR, where for decades the infectious theory and antibiotic therapy had been dismissed as heresy. Predictably, before this newest study was released to the public, the association issued a statement minimizing the positive results of earlier studies and reiterating their view of RA as an "autoimmune disease."

This time, however, attempts to contain the damage by tailoring the facts appeared to be of little or no avail. After decades of suppression, the results could no longer be denied and the focus of the media was on a possible infectious cause. An Associated Press wire story reported that the O'Dell study provided enough proof of minocycline's benefits that the drug, already in use throughout the world as a safe, effective treatment for teenage acne, soon could be widely prescribed for rheumatoid arthritis.

Even before announcement of his results, Dr. O'Dell found himself treading cautiously across a minefield of medical politics that is littered with the reputations of previous advocates of minocycline therapy and the infectious theory. Most notable among his predecessors was the late Dr. Thomas McPherson Brown, former dean of medicine at George Washington

University Medical School and director of the Arthritis Institute of the National Hospital. Dr. Brown treated some 10,000 arthritic patients with antibiotics in his fifty-year career, but despite his high success rate with the therapy, he was routinely denied access to research funds and frequently was denounced as a quack. O'Dell's research now vindicated that therapy, but stopped short of a guarantee that it would gain immediate widespread acceptance. (Brown's landmark book on his lifetime of research, *The Road Back*, is included in this volume.)

Dr. O'Dell acknowledged to a news conference at the ACR that his study included a small number of people, and he offered the familiar disclaimer that "more research is necessary." But if there was any risk that his audience might miss the point of his spectacular results, he immediately added, "However, the dramatic responses seen in our patients are important."

Although O'Dell's study was the principal seismic event at that year's ACR meeting, it wasn't the only one, and rheumatoid arthritis wasn't the only form of the disease in the new antibiotic spotlight. Another rheumatologist, Kenneth Brandt, M.D., also reported that an enzyme-inhibiting property of minocycline's sister, doxycycline, has been proven beneficial in treating osteoarthritis.

Pat Ganger, president of The Road Back Foundation, an antibiotic advocacy group named in honor of Dr. Brown's pioneering work, said of the new studies, "It is hard to believe the pharmaceutical industry will continue to ignore such an immense marketing opportunity in favor of other therapies that have already been proven to be ineffective and often toxic, simply because they yield much higher profits."

"SAFE AND EFFECTIVE . . ."

When *The Road Back* first appeared in 1988, only a handful of doctors offered the safe, inexpensive, simple antibiotic therapy for arthritis, lupus, scleroderma, or other connective tissue diseases described in Dr. Brown's book. Shortly after publication, and largely because of it, the number grew to several hundred physicians in the United States and abroad. But even as recently as the middle 1990s, some six or seven years after Brown's death, tens of thousands of other doctors—representing millions of patients—either remained unaware of the treatment or had decided to wait and see.

For those who waited, the answer was expected in the results of a study called MIRA, for Minocycline In Rheumatoid Arthritis. Under the sponsorship of the National Institutes of Health, this major clinical trial of 219 patients was conducted at study centers in New York, Vermont, Alabama, Utah, and Michigan, with the largest such group at Harvard Medical School's Beth Israel Hospital in Boston.

Patient enrollments in MIRA had begun way back in November of 1991. In a double-blind study, half the participants receive the medicine being tested, and the others get a look-alike placebo that is free of any medical properties, with neither patient nor physician knowing who gets which. The clinical portion of the trial was completed in April 1993 and the double-blind code was broken in May, but security remained so tight for the next several months that not even the physicians at the clinical centers were told how their groups had been divided. More enigmatic—and to some observers more ominous—was the fact that no provision was made for the usual follow-up with study participants after the trial was done.

The shroud on the results of the MIRA study was lifted only slightly the following November when some of the data led off that year's annual scientific meeting of the American College of Rheumatology in San Antonio. The usual vehicle for announcing medical news is a peer-reviewed journal, and in theory premature release elsewhere can jeopardize such publication. Perhaps for that reason, or perhaps because by then the politics and economics of this therapy had engendered such fierce resistance, tight controls by ACR leadership minimized the consequence of the data offered in San Antonio, and virtually none of the MIRA results found their way into the general press.

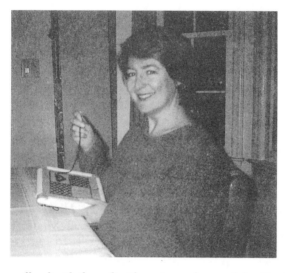

Susan Mauer, Cary, N.C., began antibiotic therapy for systemic lupus in August 1995.

I was able to kick plaquenil with no recurrence of symptoms after taking it for six years. I am deeply grateful to have been off prednisone for quite a while as well. I have none of the symptoms I suffered with the earlier therapies, and none of the side effects.

Today there are no rashes on my body, and I'm looking forward to the future again. I'm working, taking occasional evening classes, making new friends, and finding I have the energy to do things I couldn't do for years. I'm pain-free all of the time.

Recovery was slow, and it wasn't real easy. But day by day, little by little, I got better. I got my life back.

Eventually, control of those results would pass to other hands. After the preview in Texas, which was nearly a non-event, another fourteen months would elapse before the study at long last appeared in print. For the few thousand patients who had been helped by minocycline and feared that the results once again would be minimized or suppressed—which could mean future problems in finding a prescribing physician. It was a long, nervous wait. For millions more who know nothing about their disease or its treatment beyond what they hear from the Arthritis Foundation or their rheumatologists, it seems unlikely the time passed any faster just because they were left in the dark.

When the study was published at long last, it was not to an indifferent readership of rheumatologists who for years have comprised the only declining specialty in medicine, but to a constituency some forty times larger, the American College of Physicians, in its prestigious journal, *Annals of Internal Medicine*. It came out on January 15, 1995, bearing fourteen signatures, including principal investigators at the six study centers, two biostatisticians, and three physicians and research administrators from the National Institutes of Health. That many authors is bound to create the impression of a bandwagon; indeed, the entire MIRA Trial Group, including straphangers, was some five times longer, and all seventy-one of them, with their affiliations, were listed as well.

But probably the most important name was not among those attached to the study itself; it belonged to the guest author of the editorial that introduced it, Harold E. Paulus, M.D., from the UCLA School of Medicine. It was one thing for the MIRA researchers to announce that minocycline had been found to be "safe and effective" in the treatment of rheumatoid arthritis. It remained for Dr. Paulus, who had never allowed himself to be recruited to one side or the other of this highly political and often bitter controversy, to pronounce on the study's true significance.

He mentioned Tom Brown in the opening paragraph, citing his observational cohort study of ninety-eight patients in 1984 as one of the landmarks in the analysis of minocycline therapy. It set a tone. For a decade, whenever Brown's study had been cited by anyone else, it was almost inevitably accompanied by some kind of disclaimer about its scientific methodology, or worse by withering skepticism. This time there was no disclaimer, and no put-down. Instead, Dr. Paulus observed dryly that such reports had been "largely discounted because a 1971 double-blind study . . . failed to show any significant benefit from tetracycline therapy."

UNCORKING THE BOTTLE

Dr. Paulus was referring to the so-called Boston study, a tiny, poorly designed, double-blind trial of very low levels of tetracycline on a handful of RA patients at Massachusetts General

Hospital in Boston, which placed a cork in the bottle for the funding of antibiotic research that stayed tightly in place for almost a quarter century. Anyone whose faith in the scientific process remains simple and pure may find that chapter of medical history somewhat challenging, but perhaps the value of the Boston study will be in setting a useful precedent now that it has been proven wrong. If the results from only thirty patients could be embraced so ardently by those intent on proving antibiotic therapy doesn't work, then it should have been simple enough for those same enthusiasts to move to the other side of the street with flags and flowers now that other studies several times as large—and subject to far greater professional scrutiny—showed that it worked just fine.

Dr. Paulus seemed anxious to encourage such a change of heart. At San Antonio in 1993, the ACR had all but ignored a presentation by Dr. Ferdinand Breedveld and his Dutch colleagues on double-blind placebo-controlled trials in the Netherlands, and that same study got equally scant notice when it beat the MIRA report into print several months before, in 1994. In comparing them in his editorial, Dr. Paulus found the Dutch and MIRA studies "remarkably similar."

"Separately," he said, "either trial could be considered an aberration; together they must be taken seriously. Indeed, together they could be submitted to the Food and Drug Administration as the two positive 'pivotal' controlled clinical trials . . . for approval of a new drug application." He said the two studies "provide substantial evidence of the beneficial clinical effect of minocycline in patients with rheumatoid arthritis."

At least one of the clinicians in the MIRA project had entered the study expecting to confirm the negative Boston results from two decades earlier. "If tetracycline works," the widely quoted forecast went, "water works." With publication of the MIRA results, some of the forecaster's peers entertained themselves with the fancy that the same doctor, now a believer, might be preparing a grant application for clinical trials on H_2O.

The Arthritis Foundation was quick to issue its own "News Alert," with a perfunctory acknowledgment that this type of therapy had been "promoted" by the late Dr. Brown and pointing out (twice, in case readers missed it the first time) that "Minocycline is not approved by the Food and Drug Administration for the treatment of rheumatoid arthritis."

The Arthritis Foundation was certainly aware that the majority of prescriptions in America are for off-label applications and, even before the studies, FDA approval had never been required for a family doctor to prescribe minocycline for arthritis or anything else. Several months earlier the Arthritis Foundation had sold its name to Johnson & Johnson's McNeil Consumer Products Company for use on a proprietary line of high-priced aspirin, ibuprofen, and acetaminophen, an ultimately disastrous deal that *Consumer Reports* described accurately as "swapping credibility for cash." The Alert on the MIRA study strove for the familiar foundation pretense of impartiality, but to some it sounded more like marketing than medicine, one more chance to torpedo the competition for the sixty-billion-dollar American arthritis pie.

It spoke well for the NIH commitment to keeping the numbers honest that the lead author of the MIRA Study was not a rheumatologist but a prominent biostatistician, Barbara C. Tilley, Ph.D., with Henry Ford Health Systems in Detroit. The convention for the release of studies whose authors are at more than one location is for the lead author to speak for the rest and to issue the principal announcement to the press (although in this case media were referred as well to the physician at whichever of the six study centers was nearest).

"HIGHLY SIGNIFICANT IMPROVEMENTS . . ."

The headline from Detroit read, "Common Antibiotic Found Safe and Effective for Rheumatoid Arthritis"—nearly identical to the headline on the newspaper reports of O'Dell's study of this same therapy four years later. The announcement said the MIRA study was based on two theories. First, the cause of rheumatoid arthritis may be persistent infection with mycoplasma, which is known to respond to tetracycline antibiotics.

Second, minocycline blocks the enzyme process that destroys arthritic joints and modifies the inflammatory response.

The MIRA trial involved 219 adults who had rheumatoid arthritis for an average of eight years; each patient had six or more swollen joints and nine or more tender or painful joints. One group of 109 patients was given 100 milligrams of minocycline orally twice a day; the other 110 received a placebo.

"After forty-eight weeks, the study found that 54 percent of the patients taking minocycline had at least a 50 percent improvement in the number of swollen joints [and] 56 percent . . . showed at least a 50 percent improvement in the number of tender joints."

Dr. Paulus, on the other hand, didn't consider those subjective results to be anywhere nearly as noteworthy as the changes noted in the laboratory, referring to "highly significant improvement in acute-phase reactants and IgM rheumatoid factor titers, with minimal adverse events."

While none of the patients showed serious toxicity and "side effects were minimal and infrequent," seven patients did stop the therapy, most commonly for dizziness. (This is a known problem with minocycline, but apparently not with doxycyline, which Tom Brown would often use as an alternative.) The announcement then went on to compare those side effects with the current standards.

"Methotrexate (an anti-cancer drug), which is the first-line choice of treatment followed by oral gold for patients with rheumatoid arthritis, has many side effects and cannot be taken by all patients. Its side effects may include nausea, vomiting, stomach pain, diarrhea, mouth ulcers, anemia, and liver toxicity."

Another phenomenon, the so-called placebo effect where patients not receiving the treatment show improvement anyway, has always been a factor in the testing of arthritis drugs, and with MIRA it was even higher than expected. In this case, it was attributed to the fact that patients were encouraged to continue taking stable doses of NSAIDs (nonsteroidal anti-inflammatory drugs) throughout the trial. But although clinical improvement in joint swelling and tenderness began at week

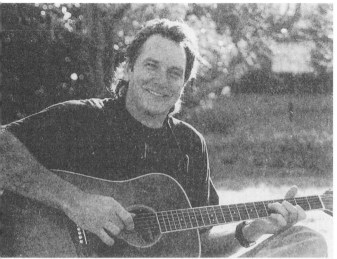

Kim Lofts, Albany, West Australia, was diagnosed with crippling rheumatoid arthritis in 1988, started antibiotic therapy in 1995, and now works on an oil-drilling platform in the South China Sea:

RA is the "Grand Thief"; it will rob you of self-esteem, dignity, pride, and life's energy. I'd lost faith in what my rheumatologist had to offer me, which came down to more drugs and no hope. Some days I was battling just to pick up my guitar, let alone play. Two years after starting antibiotics, I'm in remission. This treatment has given me a new lease on life. I'm doing things I haven't been able to do in years.

twelve for both groups, it leveled off for the placebo group in week twenty-four, while patients on minocycline continued getting better through to the end of the study.

Three days after publication of the MIRA study, an article appeared in the *Journal of the American Medical Association* on the widespread overuse of antibiotics. Antibiotic abuse, especially for relatively trivial ailments, has been a problem for years, and the *JAMA* piece focused, with good reason, on antibiotics in the penicillin family, amoxicillin and cephalosporins. For patients suffering with inflammatory forms of arthritis, the timing of the antibiotics article was devastating. While no antibiotic is entirely exempt from the potential for encouraging resistant strains of the diseases they attack, tetracyclines have long been recognized as the one class of antibiotics least subject to that disadvantage. There are several classes of common disease organisms frequently targeted by this antibiotic that have never produced a single recorded instance of a tetracycline-resistant strain. But the *JAMA* article appeared to make no such distinctions among the various types of antibiotics. Moreover, rheumatoid arthritis is hardly a trivial or transient affliction, like an earache or sinusitis. Paradoxically, the new use of minocycline for this widespread crippling disease would reverse the very trend the *JAMA* article cited as being so dangerous: the upswing of newer, more expensive, and potentially more destructive drugs—already in widespread use against RA—that can create worse problems than they ever hope to cure.

During this same period, the possibility of an infectious etiology for rheumatoid arthritis slowly began to accumulate a careful, qualified acceptance in other sectors of the scientific community. More than a year before publication of the MIRA results, a "reappraisal of the evidence that rheumatoid arthritis and several other idiopathic diseases are slow bacterial infections" appeared in *Annals of Rheumatic Diseases*. Authored by G. A. W. Rook, J. L. Stanford, and P. M. Lydyard, all with University College, London Medical School, it concluded, "The arrival of recombinant DNA technology means that the role of infections in RA . . . will be established or refuted within the next few years. If the infection hypothesis proves correct, the treatment of RA will need to be completely revised, and the consequences for the pharmaceutical industry will be enormous. It could become unethical to use steroids or agents which block prostaglandin synthesis, as we cannot be sure that they do not promote proliferation of the organism and . . . lead to more severe disease. Instead we will need to devise antibiotic regimens and immunotherapeutic protocols."

Overall, the MIRA study gave fresh impetus to this reappraisal. But if there was still a cloud hanging over the interpretation of its significance, it was in the clinical results for the placebo group. While improvements in swelling and tenderness were some 25 to 30 percent lower than in the group on minocycline, the fact that the values came even that close was, for many observers, a puzzling anticlimax.

POWER, MONEY, HEALTH

It would be difficult to overstate the importance of economics in health care. Simplicity and low cost may appear as virtues to a consumer, especially when, like minocycline or its kin in the tetracycline family, a medicine is backed by decades of safe usage in hundreds of widely varied applications. But appearances deceive: the pharmaceutical industry is not driven by the consumer, but by money.

In America alone, at least 30 million people suffer from some inflammatory form of arthritis or related connective-tissue disease, and their symptoms range from mild discomfort to agonizing incapacity. Old standards for arthritis therapy may or may not deliver short-term relief, but recent research has produced a great deal of evidence that they deliver no long-term benefits whatever. Along the way, some of them create new risks to the patient's health, and not just by allowing it to deteriorate.

One pharmaceutical firm recently sought government approval to market as an arthritis remedy a drug developed for other purposes—the common genealogy of almost every drug sold in the arthritis marketplace. When the FDA turned down the application on the grounds that the benefits were marginal and the side effects were worse than the disease, the cost of the failed gamble was $100 million. The far more expensive drugs already in wide use for arthritis generate billions of dollars in annual profits, and those profits are seriously challenged by Dr. Brown's therapy.

After the MIRA trials, even though the battle over antibiotic therapy for rheumatoid arthritis had been joined by giants, it was far from won. With its long-awaited publication, a few strong voices in the front row of the choir were at long last starting to sing Tom Brown's song, but the dissonance was still far louder than the melody. Most physicians either remained unaware of the MIRA trials or downgraded the result based on what appeared to be its high placebo effect.

THE GORDEN ANALYSIS

Some months after publication of the MIRA study, a medical statistician named Dr. Raymond L. Gorden took a closer look at the numbers. He had recently analyzed the methodology in several clinical trials of chemotherapy for cancer, and had found those studies so flawed "that no conclusions could safely be drawn except that the side effects were very damaging." Based in part on that experience, he acknowledged that he was skeptical about the "great wave of optimism among both patients and physicians" in the aftermath of such a positive report on a treatment for arthritis.

To Gorden's surprise, while he could find no fault in any of the conclusions in view of the methods used in the experiment, he did find what he described as a "serious deviation from scientific experimental design" that, although in no way detracting from the general conclusions, actually served to obscure what would have been an even more dramatic contrast between the minocycline and the placebo group in terms of joint swelling and tenderness. That serious deviation would provide the missing key to the MIRA puzzle.

The deviation he found was what the authors of the MIRA study referred to as "violations of protocol." These violations were possible because the treatment protocol was not simply that one group received minocycline and the other a placebo. Instead, out of concern for the suffering of the patients, the protocol allowed both groups some type of anti-inflammatory drug during the trial. Since those drugs have the effect of reducing joint tenderness and swelling, the very things the study was designed to measure, it was logically necessary to hold such medications at comparable levels in both groups throughout the full forty-eight weeks of the trial.

But that isn't what happened. The rules were violated 120 times during the course of the study. There were 46 violations among the 109 patients in the minocycline group, and 74 violations among the 110 patients in the placebo group. There were not only more frequent violations in the placebo group (3 out of 4 versus less than half), but 46 of those placebo group violations were for increased doses of anti-inflammatory drugs in contrast to only 19 increased doses in the minocycline group. In fact, the number of minocycline patients who *decreased* their anti-inflammatories was greater than the number who asked for more, while in the placebo the ratio was 3 to 1 in the other direction.

Gorden also pointed to a similar important difference between the two groups in the number of violations of the rule against intra-joint injections of corticosteroids: in the minocycline group there were only six such violations, in contrast to seventeen in the placebo group.

Clearly, the preponderance of violations was of the kind that would produce better results for the placebo group. Gorden next asked how the minocycline still managed to do better than the placebo despite the handicap.

The answer was that there are two ways to reduce pain and swelling in an arthritic joint. One is simply to suppress the symptoms, and the other is to reduce the cause—analogous to raising the bridge or lowering the river. Minocycline kills mycoplasma, the organism that Dr. Brown had identified as the prime suspect in RA and most other connective tissue disease as the cause of inflammation and pain. As noted, the MIRA study demonstrated that the anti-inflammatory drugs in the placebo group lost their power to further decrease the pain and swelling after the twenty-fourth week, while in the minocycline group those outer signs of the disease continued to decline through the forty-eighth week—*even though the use of anti-inflammatories by the minocycline group actually decreased during that same period.*

Gorden next asked why the attending physicians violated the protocol more frequently and more toward increases of anti-inflammatories in the placebo group than in the minocycline group. Periodic tests revealed that more placebo patients were showing worsening blood tests along with their increased joint pain and swelling. Also, thirteen in the placebo group as opposed to only two in the minocycline group dropped out because they felt no improvement or experienced an arthritic flareup. Under any of those circumstances, it seemed probable that the physician took pity on the patient and tried to reduce the symptoms by switching anti-inflammatory drugs or increasing the dosage. In other words, doctors in the study were continuing to do what they had been doing with arthritis for the past half-century: treating the symptoms instead of the disease, and then confusing the results.

"Clearly these violations of protocol and the failure to reject them from the analysis had the general effect of obscuring the actual superiority of the minocycline over the placebo," Gorden concluded. "The MIRA study does not mislead patients or physicians to overoptimistic expectations of the minocycline treatment. The minocycline was successful despite the bias against it in the performance of the experiment. Despite my original skepticism I am convinced that the MIRA study follows a valid design and therefore represents a real breakthrough in the treatment of arthritis and in the theory that the disease is caused by an infection."

NETHERLANDS, ISRAEL, BRITAIN, FRANCE: EVIDENCE ACCUMULATES

Although it has been unpopular for the past half-century, the infectious theory of rheumatoid arthritis has been around for a long time. Way back in 1920, the renowned physician Osler saw the disease as "secondary to a focus of infection," probably in the mouth and throat. Twenty years later that theory provided the initial rationale for Lande and Forestiere's successful use of gold compounds, which, though extraordinarily toxic, were known anti-microbials. This same assumption of an infectious etiology would eventually justify the use in arthritis of other drugs originally designed to fight malaria. Significantly, after the death of Dr. Brown in 1989, much of the impetus for continued revival of the infectious theory would come from abroad. The first major landmark was the publication in 1991 of an open dose-finding study of minocycline on ten Dutch patients by a researcher at Leiden University named Ferdinand Breedveld. "Half of the efficacy variables improved significantly after four weeks of therapy," the authors reported. "At the end of the study all variables were significantly changed compared with their pretreatment values. We conclude minocycline may be beneficial in RA." Even though the research was performed abroad, the results were published in the United States; it revived a rancorous controversy and instantly positioned Breedveld, a recent fellow at Harvard Medical School under Dr. David Trentham, as one of the leading investigators in antibiotic therapy.

The debate intensified the following year with publication in *Journal of Rheumatology* of another open study from abroad, this time of eighteen RA patients by a young Israeli rheumatologist named Pnina Langevitz and four colleagues in Tel Aviv. "Statistically significant improvement was noted in almost all variables of disease activity. . . . Of the twelve patients completing the study, 25 percent had complete remission, 25 percent had more than a 50 percent improvement, and the other 50 percent had moderate improvement (greater than 25 percent)." This was the first report since Brown's of actual remissions on antibiotic therapy. By now the climate in American research was so politicized, almost any research on minocycline was received by all but a few with polite curiosity, aloofness, or open disdain.

But it was an idea whose time was about to come again, and the momentum continued to accumulate. Also in 1993, a Breedveld colleague named Kloppenburg published a report in another American journal on the role of antibiotics as disease modifiers in RA, and a year later the two Leiden researchers reported in the American journal *Arthritis and Rheumatism* on the results of a far more ambitious study than Breedveld's first one. In a twenty-six-week randomized trial of eighty patients in the Netherlands with an average disease duration of thirteen years, half received 100 milligrams of minocycline orally twice a day, and the other half were given a placebo. In the minocycline group, the mean number of swollen joints decreased from 8.6 to 7.8, while in the placebo group the results went in the opposite direction, rising from 8.6 to 9.2. Similarly, scores on the Ritchie articular index for arthralgia, or joint pain, declined from 21 to 18 in the group receiving the medicine, and rose from 19 to 21 with those who didn't. "The efficacy of tetracyclines in arthritis and their limited toxicity, even when long courses are used, prompted consideration of these drugs as a possible new treatment for RA," they concluded. "The trial was performed on patients with advanced, even intractable RA. Side effects may be considered mild in relation to other established DMARDs [Disease Modifying Anti-Rheumatic Drugs]. . . . Minocycline appears to have beneficial properties in RA, even when laboratory parameters of disease activity are considered."

In 1995, an editorial on the prime infectious suspect appeared in *The Journal of Clinical Pathology*, co-authored by two key figures in European rheumatology, Dr. D. Taylor-Robinson of the Imperial College School of Medicine at St. Mary's in London, and Dr. T. Schaeverbeke of Hospital Pellegrin at the University of Bordeaux. "Mycoplasmas in rheumatoid arthritis and other human arthritides" cited numerous cases of mycoplasma-linked arthritis in rats, swine, goats, and sheep, and described a process remarkably similar to the disease in humans—including the persistence of arthritis even after the suspected trigger could no longer be recovered from the joint tissue of the infected animal. The authors commented on the successful use of polymerase chain reaction (PCR) testing, a new DNA technique for determining the role of mycoplasmas in sexually transmitted diseases, suggesting that such a test would yield important insights to the disease process if applied to patients with RA. "It is clear," they concluded, "that

Pat Ganger of Delaware Ohio, diagnosed with scleroderma in 1983, started antibiotic therapy in 1989. She is now president of The Road Back Foundation.

Systemic scleroderma does not reverse on its own, and if I hadn't read about Dr. Brown's therapy, I'm sure by now I'd be among the large majority

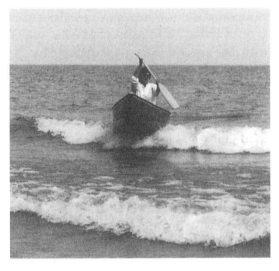

with this disease who die in the first ten years. Instead, I am in complete remission, living a full and normal life, and best of all, giving back to others.

the issue of the role of mycoplasmas in inflammatory rheumatic disorders of unknown cause, including rheumatoid arthritis, can no longer be ignored."

The reference to the possibility of future PCR testing left some of their readers with the strong suspicion that the authors were using their platform to point to the left field wall, just as Babe Ruth had sometimes done before hitting a bases-loaded homer. The suspicion was well-founded. On May 18, 1996, Taylor-Robinson, Schaeverbeke, and three other researchers reported in the British medical journal *The Lancet* on the results of their search for *Mycoplasma fermentans* in the joints of patients with RA and other forms of arthritis at Hospital Pellegrin. The infectious agent was discovered in fifteen specimens, each from a different patient, all of whom suffered from an inflammatory form of the disease. Synovial fluid was positive in 14 percent of the RA patients, and synovial tissue was positive in 40 percent, for a combined total of 21 percent of the thirty-eight RA patients in the study. Similarly, it was detected in 20 percent of the patients with spondyloarthropathy and 20 percent of those with psoriatic arthritis, and 13 percent of those with unclassified inflammatory arthritis. None of the fluid or tissue specimens was positive in the patients with reactive arthritis, JRA, osteoarthritis, post-traumatic hydrarthrosis, or gouty arthritis.

M fermentans is one of many forms of mycoplasma suspected to be implicated in arthritis over the past several decades, and the report in *The Lancet* ended with a proposal that other mycoplasmas and similar micro-organisms, particularly chlamydiae, be subjected to the same PCR examination. Placing such infectious agents at the scene is still a step away from convicting them of the crime. But far more significantly, the use of the new DNA test dramatically refuted the standard dismissal of mycoplasmas as being nothing more than laboratory contaminants.

THE NEBRASKA STUDY: 33 PERCENT REMISSIONS

One other common argument against antibiotics and the infectious theory was the persistent claim, Tom Brown and the overseas studies notwithstanding, that no credible research in the subject had ever reported remissions. Despite its benign profile and proven superiority to other DMARDs, and even despite forecasts in several of the leading journals that "the popularity of antibiotic therapy will probably accelerate" (Rheumatic Disease Clinics of North America), even today only a tiny minority of rheumatologists are willing to break ranks with ancient precedent and actually prescribe them for their patients—and then only as a last line of defense when all else fails.

Which brings us back to Dr. James O'Dell, the rheumatologist from Nebraska. O'Dell's report to the ACR in the fall of 1997 was actually the result of a three-year follow-up to a placebo-controlled clinical trial he presented as an abstract to the ACR in 1995. The study had treated minocycline as a first line of response, not a last resort, and the original abstract was clear enough about the results: O'Dell had run a multi-center study of forty-six patients with a disease duration of less than a year; 65 percent of those treated with minocycline met the high criterion of 50 percent improvement during the trial, versus a mere 13 percent for the placebo; even more conclusively, one third of the twenty-four Nebraska patients who received the minocycline were reported to have remitted during the study. Even with the reported remissions—or more likely because of them—the abstract attracted the usual response from the ACR: barely a word of the results escaped to the press, and the study was virtually buried.

Journal publication of the results was delayed for another year and a half, so the original study didn't appear in print until June of 1997, just five months before O'Dell went back to the ACR with the results of his three-year follow-up. Publication of the article attracted scant attention in the popular press that summer, trivial in proportion to its significance. All of that would change by fall, however.

On November 10, the second abstract by O'Dell and his twelve co-authors was released to the public. The ACR disclaimer that accompanied it to the press was redolent with the familiar pattern of revisionism and faint praise: in setting the context, for example, the release described as "modest" the results of the earlier MIRA and Netherlands studies, apparently in the belief that the world would have forgotten by then that those same results previously were described by Paulus and others as "profoundly significant." Dr. Doyt Conn of the Arthritis Foundation said the earlier studies had in fact discouraged many physicians from using the therapy.

The Associated Press article by medical writer Lauran Neergaard gave a perfunctory nod to the ACR disclaimers, then went right to the heart of the story: "How long improvement lasted was key, because many other treatments either wear off or eventually cause serious side effects. So O'Dell followed his patients for over three years—and 44 percent ultimately improved by a dramatic 75 percent or more."

In the follow-up, the patients he tracked were the fifteen responders to the minocycline therapy in the initial trial. By the end of the three years, five were still in complete remission. Another five were improved by the extremely high criterion of 75 percent. Two were experiencing efficacy but with some minor side effects. Three were currently on DMARDs or prednisone. All fifteen responders had been followed for a mean of 3.3 years, and all of them flared after minocycline was stopped, some within two weeks, others after as long as two and a half years; thirteen of the fifteen responded to the restarting of the antibiotic.

As he had three years before, O'Dell warned against assuming from the dramatic remission rate that the therapy was a cure, or even that rheumatoid arthritis was now proven to be an infectious disease; he theorized that the minocycline worked at least in part not just as an antibiotic but by blocking the enzymes that destroy cartilage inside joints.

The AP quoted a Minneapolis rheumatologist named Dr. Eric Schned who described O'Dell's results as "impressive" and said he had begun prescribing "safe and quite gentle" doses of minocycline to his own patients. "I tell them, 'Look, this could be a very slow medicine in working, but you may have some significant benefit extending a few years out.'"

Even the Arthritis Foundation's spokesman conceded that this time the results with minocycline showed "a very definite improvement"—but only after reminding the reader of the "small" patient base.

In fact, the Nebraska trial was half again as large as the Boston study, which with the aegis of the Arthritis Foundation had been considered more than ample to seal the fate of antibiotic therapy for a generation.

SCLERODERMA: THE HARVARD STUDY

In 1995, The Road Back Foundation funded a pilot study at Beth Israel/Deaconess Hospital, Harvard Medical School, of minocycline in scleroderma. Although not a form of arthritis, scleroderma is in the same family of connective tissue diseases, and offered a potentially dramatic model for the efficacy of minocycline therapy. Because of its systemic nature it is most frequently treated by a rheumatologist and, in the systemic form, is usually fatal. There was no universally accepted treatment for the disease.

Seven years before, when Dr. Brown described in *The Road Back* the results he achieved with minocycline therapy in scleroderma, one of his readers was Pat Ganger. After her treatment and recovery, Pat founded The Road Back Foundation, and she later shared her story with Dr. Trentham, who was already familiar with similar anecdotal evidence from Brown's book. Dr. Trentham started some scleroderma patients of his own on the therapy, and was impressed with the results, so when Pat returned with a proposal he welcomed the chance to conduct a trial.

The clinical portion of the study was completed in the spring of 1997, and by mid-November Trentham's office produced a draft report entitled *Minocycline in Early Diffuse Scleroderma: A Pilot Open 12-Month Study in 11 Patients.*

The report said that all other medications that might potentially modify scleroderma (whether or not they ever had) were discontinued during the course of the study and required a one-month washout period; such agents included methotrexate, penicillamine, chlorambucil, cyclosporin, cyclophosphidamide, colchicine, and photophoresis.

Skin biopsies were performed on all patients at enrollment. All visits included a complete history, physical examination, complete blood count, electrolytes, urea and creatinine, liver function tests, erythrocyte sedimentation rate (ESR Westergren method), and urinalysis. Serum was also collected at all visits for adhesion molecule assays.

Skin scores were measured at each visit, and a response was not counted as clinically significant unless it showed a decrease of more than 35 percent by the last examination. The researchers used a patient and physician 10-cm visual analog scale to measure global patient status, where 0 cm meant the patient could not be better, and 10 cm could not be worse; a clinically significant response was defined as a decrease of at least 25 percent in twelve months.

All eleven patients in the study had been diagnosed by at least one independent rheumatologist.

At the end of the year, five patients had dropped out of the study, two because of a renal crisis (from the disease, not the drug) just two months after entry, two for non-compliance with the protocol, and one because of death from a pre-existing cancer that was not detected until after the study began. In the two cases of renal crisis, neither was taking angiotension-converting enzyme inhibitors during the study; afterward, one returned to normal while the other required permanent dialysis. One of the two non-compliers stopped minocycline after nine months because she felt it wasn't working, although her skin score at six

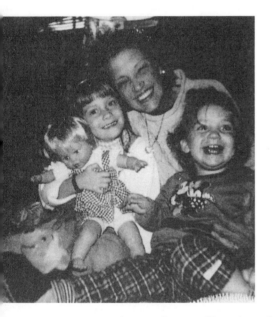

Marge Cortegiano, Long Island, N.Y., suffered with lupus, RA, and Sjogrens. After such prior medications as gold, cytoxan, plasmapheresis, and seventeen years of prednisone, she was so weak that her muscles atrophied.

After just a year on antibiotic therapy, I am incredibly grateful for the progress I have made. I am able to drive, do errands, pay my bills, travel, and play with my grandchildren (pictured)—all previously impossible because of the pain and fatigue. I keep trying new things; I just went ice skating for the first time in years to build up my muscles. The minocin has given me a whole new outlook.

months was 60 percent better than at enrollment. The other non-complier quit the study in order to switch over to intravenous minocycline therapy. Three of the dropouts were due to serious intercurrent morbidity.

Six patients completed the full course of treatment.

In all, nine of the eleven patients in the study (82 percent) experienced significant improvement in skin scores. At the end of one year, four of them had complete resolution of their skin disease and their final skin scores were zero; in three of those four, patient and physician VAS scores had improved to zero as well.

Nothing else ever came close to that kind of result.

The Harvard study will be presented to a peer-reviewed medical forum coincidentally with the publication of this book.

A PATIENT'S NEED TO KNOW

Prescriptions are written by doctors, not by their patients, and until physicians are confronted by educated consumers, there is very little incentive for them to change.

After years of misdirected research and suppression of creative dissent, fundamental new insights are now available to arthritis and its treatment. But just because MIRA therapy repeatedly has been proven effective doesn't mean physicians will automatically give it to everyone it can help. In some cases, that will depend on how effectively arthritis patients are able to use the power in this new knowledge.

That is the reason for this book.

PART I
WAITING FOR MIRA

Cornerstone

D r. Thomas McPherson Brown was eighty-two years old when *The Road Back* was first published in 1988. Joan Lunden on "Good Morning America" introduced him as the author of a book on rheumatoid arthritis that was turning the American medical establishment upside down. Ronald Reagan was in Moscow that morning and the report of the president's trip had occupied most of the program, so this segment was being squeezed into the final two minutes of the show. It was Dr. Brown's first appearance on live national television, and as he was being led out to the cameras, one of the studio personnel had advised him in a whisper to keep his answers short and sharp—that his effectiveness in making his case would be measured in fractions of a second. Despite that warning, for a moment Dr. Brown cocked his head quizzically, as though the introduction had caught him by surprise and needed weighing. Then he nodded, smiled somewhat puckishly, and said, "If that's what the book is doing, that would be a good thing."

A few yards away in the greenroom (where guests wait before being brought out to the cameras), three of his friends were anxiously watching the monitor. It was only when we all tentatively let out our breaths at the same time that I realized how apprehensive we had been for him. We all knew Dr. Brown was dying, and just minutes before he entered the set he had been seized by a fit of coughing so severe he had become violently ill. It seemed miraculous that he was able to speak at all, much less to recover the poise and humor to defend himself and his theory before an immense, nationwide audience. There was no question where he found his strength. Tom Brown knew that this was his last major opportunity to explain his book, a labor of love written in what he knew at the start was likely to be the final year of his life. Even his detractors agreed that at the very least *The Road Back* defined his position as an important medical heretic. It just wasn't in his character to quit such a long race when he seemed so close to the finish line.

In response to friendly, gentle questioning from anchor Lunden, Dr. Brown described the two central concepts in the book. After the introduction, his answers sounded disarmingly simple. The first was that every inflammatory, or rheumatoid, form of arthritis starts with an infection. The second was that all those rheumatoid forms can be treated effectively with safe, easy, and inexpensive antibiotic therapy. At that time, however, neither Dr. Brown's infectious theory nor his approach to therapy agreed with accepted views of this ancient disease.

The camera shifted to another, much younger physician, who was introduced as a spokesman for the American Rheumatism Association. Although the second introduction omitted to mention that Thomas McPherson Brown had helped found the ARA several decades earlier, for those who were aware of it there was high drama in the pending confrontation. Just a few weeks before, the ARA had attacked Brown's book, claiming that his theory and his treatment had already been scientifically disproven and suggesting that they were possibly dangerous.

The confrontation hardly lived up to its prologue. The younger doctor was cordial and spoke to Dr. Brown with respect; his tone seemed more collegial, even supportive, than challenging. The discussion seemed too abstract to engage the average viewer, and the show closed with the ARA spokesman saying that Dr. Brown and he agreed more than they disagreed. As revolutions go—especially in comparison with what was happening that morning in Moscow—it was a distinct anti-climax. But for the friends who were watching from the green-room, the end of the program brought a collective sigh of relief. When Dr. Brown returned to us, his administrative assistant, Carla Denton, threw her arms around his shoulders and kissed his cheek, and I saw tears brimming in her eyes. After the rest of us shook his hand and congratulated him on his presentation, I glanced over at the physician from the ARA, who had packed his papers and was about to leave the room alone. "You should have someone to congratulate you as well," I said, holding out my hand. "I know we're on opposite sides, but you did a good job."

He accepted the handshake, "I could have been tougher" he said, then lowered his voice. "But I didn't expect to find him in this condition."

Behind him, Dr. Brown was now seating himself slowly on one of the plastic-covered greenroom chairs. His skin was yellow, there was perspiration on his forehead, and his hands were shaking as he sipped at a cup of water that Carla was helping him hold. He looked smaller than ever, and in these past few days, for the first time since I had known him, I realized how fragile he had become. "He was afraid he wasn't going to be able to see it through," I said.

The doctor had not released the handshake, and now he grasped my elbow with his other for emphasis: "This isn't just a cough. Dr. Brown is very, very sick."

A moment later, the ARA doctor's taxi arrived and he went his separate way. At almost the same time a limo was brought around to take the rest of us back to the airport. The driver made one stop at a nearby hotel for Carla to check out. Meanwhile, in the car, Dr. Brown's head tilted slowly forward until his chin rested on his chest, and when I asked him a question he didn't answer. He stirred at a touch on his arm, but it was clear he was fighting unconsciousness. Carla returned and we debated whether to continue to the airport, but Dr. Brown raised his head and waved the conversation to an end with a small gesture of his hand. He said in a firm voice that he was just resting, and that he wanted to get home.

At LaGuardia, he seemed to be improved, although he still appeared to be unsteady on his feet. He managed to reach the gate to board the plane with helpers on each arm, and I asked one last time if he was going to be all right. He paused to weigh the question, just as he had an hour earlier on television, and then he gave the same tired but clear-eyed smile. "I'll be fine," he said "I did what I came for."

Looking back, that makes a pretty good summary of his life.

ON BEING RIGHT AT THE WRONG TIME

Dr. Brown's notoriety did not begin with the publication of the book. By the time I met him he had been defending his view of arthritis for the better part of a half century. By 1988, however, the compass that guides scientific research in rheumatology—after decades of pointing in the opposite direction—was slowly and begrudgingly starting to shift back to the infectious theory. For the majority of his professional career, Dr. Brown had been forced to dine on a heretic's standard fare, which ranged from polite tolerance to open ridicule. But by the time he decided to write the book, a small number of other researchers in the field were, at long last, openly discussing the likelihood that inflammatory arthritis had an infectious etiology, even if there still wasn't much support for the notion that it could be cured. And many more suspected, at the very least, that up to then they had been looking in the wrong place.

For forty years, that wrong place had been in a never-never land of endocrinology. In retrospect, it is easy enough to see how the research effort had been diverted. In the 1940s, a doctor at the Mayo Clinic made medical history with the isolation of one of the body's most important steroids, cortisone. Even in the Golden Age of wonder drugs, cortisone seemed nearly miraculous. The hormone suppresses inflammation, and it proved so effective in temporarily relieving the symptoms of the rheumatoid forms of arthritis that some of its advocates began to claim it as a cure.

They were right about the temporary relief, but they couldn't have been more wrong about the cure. A cure works by attacking causes, while cortisone is limited entirely to the masking of effects. With a painful disorder like arthritis, even short-term relief can be a blessing. But there are limits to the amount of cortisone a body can tolerate, and for how long. In heavy doses, its use eventually has to be terminated or terrible things will happen, including blindness and death. When the steroids are stopped, the symptoms almost always return more viciously than before.

Today most doctors, though not all, know the limits of steroids and use them sparingly to good effect. But the early excitement over cortisone set a pattern of erroneous assumptions and false expectations from which the field of rheumatology has yet to recover. By the time the fallacy became widely recognized, the U.S. government had committed an immense amount of funding for research in symptomatic therapy—not for appropriate short-term relief, but as medicine's first and often final defense against the disease. The resulting detour to symptomatic relief that began with cortisone eventually became one of the best lighted, most heavily traveled dead-end streets in the history of modern medicine.

Far worse than its cost outright, the commitment to this dead end consumed almost every resource available. Basic research into the older concept of rheumatoid arthritis as an infectious disease was almost completely abandoned in the shift to cortisone. For nearly half a century it eclipsed the infectious theory as the avenue to understanding the basic mechanism of arthritis and to its eventual cure.

The persistence of the folly that led to that long detour owes to more than bad science; it also evolved from a familiar combination of politics and money. All ideas, good or bad, need champions to support them, and the champions who aligned the arthritis-research establishment behind cortisone for half a century set about their advocacy by systematically sweeping the field of opposition. Tom Brown was a champion as well, but he was at a terrific disadvantage: nearly alone in the willingness to defend his theory and treatment, the target of ridicule and political vengeance for his opposition to misuse of cortisone, and handicapped by ethical misgivings about double-blind studies; even when he tried to overcome those misgivings, the NIH peer review system consistently refused to support his research. Good science permits dissent; in fact, dissent is the only road to discovery and change. The most damaging legacy of the cortisone advocates was that during their ascendancy it became extremely dangerous to disagree with the new dogma. For several long decades, except for Thomas McPherson Brown, who was regarded by many as the last nut on the tree, the kind of creative dissent that produces change virtually disappeared.

From a strictly business standpoint, that wasn't such a bad thing. The most lucrative diseases for the medical community are the ones that can be treated indefinitely without being cured; and each year arthritis medicines produce billions of dollars in profits for pharmaceutical companies. Although not a single one of these drugs was developed specifically to cure arthritis, chronic disease is a $600 billion gold mine in America alone, and arthritis accounts for 10 percent of that treasure.

Most of the drugs were produced initially to fight something else, like cancer or malaria, and the rest are copies that produce parallel effects without violating the original patents. Because the metabolic approach was wrong at its core, the majority of the so-called "arthritis drugs" are aimed at the symptoms with only an occasional nod to the possible cause. Hundreds of millions of public dollars—managed by administrators whose careers almost all began under the patronage or employment of the same pharmaceutical firms whose compounds they were now screening—were spent in testing and passing these new applications.

As a result, there are few areas of medicine with a lower cure rate than rheumatology or, until recently, a drearier record of basic scientific progress. The Arthritis Foundation, the nearest organization to a patient-advocacy group in this field, never tires of warning the public that the cause of rheumatoid arthritis is unknown, that it cannot be cured, and that patients must direct their energies toward learning how to live with their affliction. Whatever its intention, when the most common way of dealing with failure is to shove it all back on the patient and blame a poor attitude, the strategy is bound to make the disease even harder, not easier, for the arthritic.

It's also harder for the doctor, and rheumatology can be a frustrating, unrewarding choice for physicians whose principal purpose in life is to heal the sick. Although some rheumatologists earn incomes of half a million dollars or more a year, the field is considered to be a low-paying one. Perhaps more important, arthritis specialists lack many of the spiritual rewards found in most fields of medicine, and the specialty is declining. At best, the doctor can hope to hold the line long enough for the patient to go into spontaneous remission; sometimes it happens, more often it doesn't.

In common with many branches of clinical medicine, rheumatology offers few rewards for innovation. Real cures may be a rarity, but doctors don't lose malpractice suits if they can prove they followed the traditional path, and there's substantial risk for the physician who openly departs from established procedure. For forty years, that's been the basic Catch 22 of the infectious theory, and in particular of antibiotic therapy: the rewards are not for success but for failure, and the only penalty is for advocating basic change.

Today, at long last, the medical perspective on the causes and treatment of inflammatory arthritis has begun to broaden, and the pressure for change can no longer be denied. When Tom Brown and I first met to write the book that would become his legacy, any omens of a coming revolution were still so tentative and vague as to be all but invisible. Since then, however, the horizon gradually brightened, and more recently had been filled with signs and wonders. One of the earliest such wonders came in May of 1992, just three years after Tom Brown's death

and four years after the publication of his book, when enrollment was completed for NIH-backed clinical trials of the efficacy of the antibiotic therapy described in *The Road Back*.

Dr. Brown might have been uncomfortable that it was a
double-blind study, but without a doubt he would have been
delighted that there was any study at all. Double-blind meant
that half of the subjects would receive the medication being
tested—in this case, the tetracycline minocycline—and the
other half got a pill that had no medical properties at all. The
testing centers were Beth Israel Hospital in Boston, University
of Vermont in Burlington, State University of New York in
Brooklyn, Henry Ford Hospital in Detroit, University of Utah
Medical Center in Salt Lake City, and University of Alabama in
Birmingham.

WHAT HAPPENED NEXT

The NIH clinical trials set the stage for a seismic shift in the
basic approach to treatment. Even though these changes
promised to revolutionize a major branch of medicine, none of
them required any amendment to Tom Brown's view of the disease as he described it in the book from his own research and
lifelong clinical experience. (*The Road Back* is included in this
volume.)

Despite the terrible burden of unproven truth that Brown
carried with him through his life, his friends, colleagues, and
patients never knew him to be bitter. He loved his patients,
even—and perhaps especially—the ones he knew he would
never see, and right up to the end he suffered his detractors
with a Quaker stoicism that frequently impressed his less for-
bearing co-author as saintly.

Some of that stoicism may have been catching. Even before
the MIRA trials, many of Dr. Brown's patients who had initially
viewed the book as their and his final chance to win over the
medical community had slowly come to accept the possibility
that their hopes might still be fulfilled, but not within their
deliverer's lifetime. It was commonplace to hear at the outset of

the book project that if Dr. Brown didn't live long enough to see this through—including total capitulation by the opposition—then it couldn't possibly happen after he was gone. A year and a half later, some of those same people recognized that the process was a lot slower than they had hoped, but there was no doubt something had been started and was gathering momentum. Even then, however, no one could know how long it would last or where it was to lead.

One evening in mid-April 1989, I walked out to the office behind my house on Cape Cod and called Tom Brown at the National Hospital. It was a familiar pattern for both of us; the best time to reach him was at the end of evening rounds when his work day was almost over. The difference was that this time he was a patient in that hospital, and we both knew there was a good chance the call would be our final conversation. We traded small talk for a moment or two, and then I asked him if he was terribly disappointed that the book had not yet lived up to Joan Lunden's prophecy of a year before.

There was a pause, and I could picture him cocking his head, clear-eyed as ever, to weigh the question. "I never thought of myself as turning the medical world upside down; if anything, I was trying to set it rightside up," he said. Despite the fatigue and the difficulty in speaking, his voice was still warmed by the familiar smile. "The way this is turning out, it looks like you're the one who'll learn whether I succeeded. But there's one thing I know I managed to do for the medical world, just because I wouldn't give up and go away: I've succeeded in giving it one terrific, fifty-year pain in the neck. That's got to be worth something."

I agreed it was. We were both still laughing when we said good-bye.

CHAPTER 2.

A Ten-Foot Pole

The first time I ever heard of Thomas McPherson Brown, I was lying in a rope hammock hung between two ocean-edge palm trees at Caribe Playa on the southeast coast of Puerto Rico. There may be something about being on vacation, about being suspended far from responsibility or consequence, that encourages a false sense of immunity from fate. I had no idea how that moment would change my life.

It was in the early spring of 1987. A couple named Jane and Alan Fagan were staying in the next room to ours, near the end of the row in the oceanfront hotel. The Fagans came from just outside Boston, and in the course of trading the usual data we found that Alan and I had been to the same high school and college, and that we had a number of mutual friends. They were ideal vacation neighbors: energetic but laid back, obviously more than satisfied with each other's company and careful not to intrude on our short time there, but full of good information when we asked for it, on local happenings, places to eat, sights to see. Best of all, they shared a wonderfully sly sense of humor, and we all found something to laugh about every time we ran into them.

They appeared to be in their early sixties. Alan, trim and patrician, had recently retired as head of a secretarial school in Boston. Jane, elegantly petite and constantly smiling, was a painter. They said they spent part of each summer in Nova Scotia, where she had grown up as the granddaughter of a provincial senator. Early on, Jane revealed that she had suffered for years from crippling rheumatoid arthritis.

Jane asked me what I wrote; when I said mostly about business and medicine, she raised her eyebrows and smiled mysteriously—"Aha!"—and in her eyes the bobbins set to spinning. It was later that same day that she came over to the hammock and told me about Dr. Brown.

The way she did it was charming, circumspect, engaging. But writers are approached almost daily by people with agendas, and I suspected instantly she was trying to sell me something. I tried to be just as casual and charming right back, on some other subject. The last thing in the world I wanted to hear about on a four-day vacation was rheumatoid arthritis. Jane gracefully followed me to the new topic. She was disarmingly good at allowing herself to be deflected—so good, in fact, I even thought afterward that maybe I had been wrong about her intention. I had a lot to learn from the senator's granddaughter.

Ten days after our return to Cape Cod, I was back at my desk in the carriage house when the telephone rang. "Hello, neighbor," said a sunny, lilting voice that I recognized instantly as belonging to Unit Two. She told me she was calling from her bed in the National Hospital for Orthopedics and Rehabilitation just outside Washington.

"What happened?" I asked. "What are you doing there?"

"Why would you ask a question like that?" she said, pretending to scold me. "I'm here to see Dr. Brown, of course. For my arthritis."

I tried to recall what she had started to tell me that day when I had been floating in the hammock by the gentle breakers of Caribe Playa. Dr. Brown had some kind of treatment. Or was it a theory? But the only thing that came to mind with any clarity was the image of her small, soft hands, the pale, gnarled fingers turned sideways from their metacarpals like rain-bent reeds, and the recollection of having wondered, when I first saw them, where she still found the strength to hold a brush or palette.

I also recalled my earlier sense of an agenda, and this time I realized she was not to be deterred.

"Maybe it would be better if you started again," I said.

She did.

Jane Fagan was my first case history on rheumatoid arthritis. She had had it for years, and as almost always happens it had gotten progressively worse, to the point where her doctors in the best hospitals in Boston gave up on her. "They told me I'd be in a wheelchair by now, and if I'd listened to them, that's just where I'd be. If you get involved in this, you'll hear that story over and over again. It makes me just boiling mad, but for most people that's the way this disease ends, in a wheelchair or a bed or the cemetery, once their doctors decide their bodies can't stand the battle and it's over. Instead, thank God, I found Dr. Brown."

She then went on about her rescuer, reciting his credentials: Chairman of the Arthritis Institute of the National Hospital, former Chairman of the Department of Medicine of George Washington University, a medical consultant to the White House, and so on. I kept thinking about all the reasons I didn't want to write about rheumatoid arthritis, but every time one of them came to mind, Jane rolled out a new chapter of his résumé or the story of another patient whose life had been restored by Dr. Brown's treatment, and I found myself teetering back and forth, disengaging and then caught up again.

I finally interrupted her. Of all the disorders in medicine, it was hard to think of a single one more fraught with peril; the subject was a sinkhole for any lay writer hoping to be taken seriously. More outright quackery had been written about rheumatoid arthritis, for a longer time, than any other condition on earth.

"That's another thing," she cut back in, undaunted, "it's not a condition. Diabetes is a condition. Rheumatoid arthritis is a disease." She then explained the analog to diabetes and the consequences that had followed from the isolation of cortisone in the late 1940s. "All the drugs that have come since do pretty much the same thing," she went on. "In one way or another, they mask the symptoms. Up to a point, that's good. But if the doctor relies on nothing else, while the arthritis may look like it's getting better, it's actually getting worse." There wasn't the slightest trace of doubt in her tone, and I smiled at how much tougher she was on the telephone than she had ever been in Puerto Rico. The only defense was to be tough right back. "I'd rather write about Elvis sightings or flying saucers. If Dr. Brown's theory or treatment is so terrific, why doesn't he write about it himself?"

Over the years, she answered calmly, he had published more than a hundred articles and papers in medical and scientific periodicals. But far more important than that, he had treated some 10,000 patients, and almost all of them had gotten better. Dr. Brown was very careful not to call his treatment a cure, but a lot of his patients called it just that "because it often is," she said with certitude. What he needed—what his theory and treatment needed—was someone who could translate the things Dr. Brown had done and the things he had written into a language that could be understood by everybody. Jane asked if I knew how many people suffer from this disease.

"Lots." The vise was tightening.

"In the millions." There was a short pause, but still plenty of time to translate that vast, unspecified population into imagined readers. "Millions and millions," she added, perhaps a bit wickedly, for emphasis.

By way of response, I allowed myself a wary laugh.

She countered with a resigned, discouraged-sounding sigh, almost as though she were giving up, and said plaintively, "I thought it was something you might write for the *Reader's Digest*."

"I've never written for the *Reader's Digest*, but I can't imagine they'd touch this with a ten-foot pole. If this theory and treatment were valid, they'd have done the story already. And for that matter, doctors all over the world would be using Brown's approach, instead of whatever it is they're doing."

"Well, it needs so much explaining—" she said, leaving the thought unfinished because she knew that explaining is what writers do for a living. "Besides, that isn't the way things work in medicine—there's such resistance to change. It's a lot safer for doctors to kill their patients with treatments that have been approved than to cure them with ones that challenge tradition."

It was obvious Jane knew that writers like to think of themselves as solvers of problems and untanglers of plots. Perhaps I would imagine myself an Alexander, confronting this Gordian knot with a sword of words. "The complexity may be part of the problem," I said, half aware of the risk that she might mistake my caution for interest. "It sounds less like an article than a book."

"A book!" She was coming back to life again, and I nearly bit my tongue. When I assured her it was not a book I was proposing to write, she asked, "Would you consider talking to Dr. Brown by telephone?"

To my surprise, I heard myself say, "Why not?" but with a quick codicil: "I'm not going to call him—because I don't want to mislead him into thinking I'm looking for a story. If he's at all interested, then you can give him my number."

Jane thanked me. We traded some laughs about our time in Puerto Rico, and I wished her well. We made vague plans for all of us getting together for a reunion, in Boston or on the Cape, once she was finished at the hospital. There was never any doubt in my mind that arthritis is a cruel, painful, lonely disease, and I hoped our conversation had satisfied her need to be heard. But that was the end of it; how could she ever persuade Dr. Brown to pick up the telephone and call someone he'd never met?

I would never learn the answer, but he called at nine o'clock that night, right after finishing his evening rounds.

Over the telephone, Thomas McPherson Brown was everything Jane had said he was. He was warm, friendly, witty, and, above all, straightforward. In response to questions about his long, distinguished career, when he came to the part about the opposition he had encountered with his theory and treatment, he answered without the slightest hint of rancor or polemics. He had not originated the infectious theory; it had been around for decades. And he had hardly invented the treatment; tetracycline was one of the oldest antibiotics and one of the most thoroughly tested, an obvious choice for treating a wide variety of infections. However, he admitted he may have been the first to put the theory and treatment together in the field of rheumatology.

A big part of the controversy about his view of rheumatoid arthritis, he said, was related to something called mycoplasma, a microorganism without cell walls that was halfway between bacteria and viruses. Nearly fifty years earlier, as a young physician conducting medical research at the Rockefeller Institute in New York, he had isolated these germs from the joint fluid of a woman with rheumatoid arthritis, and he suspected they could be the infectious cause of her disease. It wasn't an easy trick; mycoplasma is extremely elusive, and Brown had tried unsuccessfully a couple hundred times before he found what he was looking for.

Meanwhile, down the hall from his lab, a young colleague named Albert Sabin was searching for the answer to infantile paralysis. Knowing of Brown's work, one day he extracted some tissue from an arthritic mouse and injected it in another mouse who was disease-free. When the second mouse came down with arthritis, Sabin passed along the results to Brown. A short time later, at about the same time the Nazi armies swept into Poland, the *New York Times* published a long story on the possibility that Tom Brown's isolation of mycoplasma might be a medical breakthrough.

The Second World War interrupted everything, but afterward, when other researchers tried once or twice and failed to duplicate the results Brown had achieved only after many attempts, they dismissed his findings as a mistake, saying the mycoplasmas he claimed to have isolated must have been contaminants. Then cortisone came into the picture, and the medical world stopped listening.

By the 1980s, other researchers using new techniques were able to isolate mycoplasmas from arthritic joint fluid almost routinely. This tardy vindication of Brown's early claim may have been gratifying intellectually and scientifically, but it still didn't prove the cause of the disease. Besides, although he didn't say it in so many words, perhaps Tom Brown knew by then he had been standing too long outside the gate, and it was too late to redeem his reputation as a heretic.

Just about everyone who is attracted to unpopular causes, especially in medicine, is familiar with the story of Hungarian physician Ignaz Phillip Semmelweis and his long, heartbreaking crusade to prove that another widespread disease, puerperal fever, was infectious. In many ways, the story seemed to parallel the odyssey of Thomas McPherson Brown. In one year in Berlin, the infection of childbirth fever was so rampant that not a single mother or infant involved in a hospital delivery survived more than a week after childbirth. Semmelweis said puerperal fever was actually cadaveric poisoning, transferred to the mother and child during examinations or delivery by the doctor's unwashed hands. It was not until long after his death in 1865 that the theory was finally accepted, and generations of infanticide by the fatal touch of the delivering physician came to an end.

In listening to Dr. Brown, the prospect of a once-in-a-lifetime opportunity to do good was more than balanced by the sense of enormous risk. The danger was not so much from the possibility that he was wrong; that issue could be resolved by talking with a lot more of his patients. Even if he was right, however, any challenge to conventional wisdom, especially one as tangible as a book, was bound to incense even further those who still condemned him.

From that first conversation, it was apparent Tom Brown was a natural teacher, and in one respect, at least, the book would be an easy one to write. When I shared my misgivings about tackling such a controversial subject, he quickly agreed: "As a writer, you'd be taking a chance." I waited for the disclaimer but there was none, and that, too, was persuasive. We agreed to think it over.

We spoke several times in the next few days, and with his encouragement I began calling some of his present and former patients. Half of them wept with gratitude when they described what he had done for them, and almost everyone said he had saved them from pain and improved their lives. Looking back on it, that wasn't what I wanted to hear; it would have been so much easier to walk away from all of this if I had been able to shrug him off, after due diligence on my part, as being simply misguided. We both knew he was being selective in the names he gave me, so to avoid the chance he was salting the mine I asked for a list of all the patients he had ever treated at the Arthritis Institute. When the names were called at random, the results were the same.

By the end of that process, it was clear that Tom Brown was exactly what Jane Fagan had said he was: a great healer who possessed an extraordinary gift—not just of character or skill, but a gift of knowledge that had to be shared with the world.

A week later, I sent my agent a proposal for a book titled *The Road Back: Rheumatoid Arthritis—Its Cause and Its Treatment*, by Thomas McPherson Brown, M.D., and Henry Scammell. Despite what Tom Brown had said about risk, it was obvious that most of the peril was for him rather than for me. He was the physician and it was his story; my role was simply to supply some of the language.

Three weeks later, the agent called to say he had found a publisher. Elated, I called Washington. I'll never forget Tom Brown's response when I told him the news. He laughed with delight, and then he asked me if I was scared.

It seemed an odd question, and instead of answering it, I told him I was certain we were about to make history.

"I hope so," he said. "But I also hope you know what you're letting yourself in for. I've been at this a long time, and some things don't change as easily as others. In medicine, when you challenge the way people think about what they've been doing—especially what they've been doing wrong—you're certain to find yourself with a whole lot of opposition."

CHAPTER 3

Landmarks

W e met in Washington a few days after accepting the publisher's offer. Although it was our first meeting face to face, we had long since developed an easy familiarity from the hours of telephone conversations and, not surprisingly, Tom Brown turned out to be every bit as warm and welcoming in person. What did prove surprising were his tremendous energy and youthfulness.

At the most, he appeared to be in his late sixties, all the more astonishing for the fact that he had been fighting prostatic cancer for the previous five years. He was short, and he still walked with a cane after recent hip surgery related to the disease having migrated to the bone. When I asked him about his health, he said he tired easily but that the cancer was under control; the response was friendly and seemed direct enough, but it didn't invite further query. Even though he moved slowly, I found myself thinking of him more as a tennis player, which he told me had been his favorite recreation until the cancer, and not at all as a victim.

In the two intense years between that meeting and his death, there would never be a single moment when Tom Brown gave the slightest hint that he thought of himself as a victim of anything.

We met a few hours each day for several days in a row on that first visit, and I listened with a tape recorder as he worked his way through the outline we had developed for the first few chapters. I was impressed that even when I probed deeply for personal details of the problems he encountered, especially during the early days when the rejection of his peers must have been most painful, his responses remained remarkably disciplined and free of rancor. Never once did he digress into the kind of self-justification, complaining, or recrimination that would have been irresistible to a lesser man who had lived through the same ordeal. He had no intention of using this project as a forum to settle old scores.

As the book took shape, I returned to Washington several times in the following months, and on one of those trips Tom made arrangements for me to visit the National Museum of Natural History at the Smithsonian Institution, where an old friend and Johns Hopkins classmate, Dale Stewart, was the director emeritus. The visit was based on the hope that the human skeletal remains in the museum's collections might supply some clue to the anthropological history of rheumatoid arthritis, and possibly to its infectious etiology. Up to that time no scientific method had been developed to distinguish between joint damage from disease during life and the effects of postmortem erosion, but medical detectives hoped that part of the answer might be hidden in the museum collection. At minimum, becoming known at the Smithsonian would increase the chance of hearing about such a development if it finally happened.

Dr. Stewart's office was on the third floor, a part of the museum that is closed to the public. When the elevator door opened, the long passageway ahead seemed to disappear into shadows. The walls were lined on both sides with floor-to-ceiling cabinets or stacks of wide, dark green drawers. It was a sweltering day, but the dimly lit corridors had a sense of cool timelessness. On finally reaching Stewart's office he revealed that the files were actually a carefully indexed cemetery; the drawers contained the skeletal remains of more than 33,000 people. After a short conversation and tour around the laboratories, Dr. Stewart introduced his successor as department head, a tall, serious Kansan less than half his age named Douglas Ubelaker. Dr. Ubelaker said he was familiar with some of the anthropological research on arthritis then under way, and he promised to keep us in mind if any of it produced results. That promise proved to be a valuable one.

In the course of the next several weeks I met dozens of Tom Brown's patients and interviewed many of them in depth for the case histories we would use in the book. Our organizational plan was to alternate chapters that explained the science with chapters that traced the history of the disease through individual lives. One of the pitfalls in dealing with medicine is that the scientific issues can become so abstract the reader loses any sense of human consequence, and Tom Brown was determined not to let that happen.

We knew the decision to include cases carried a risk on the other side as well: in arthritis, medical researchers are quick to dismiss such "anecdotal evidence," a term that for some invokes the image of liars sitting around a cracker barrel. But in clinical rheumatology as in any other branch of medicine, the patient's self-assessment is one of the most valuable tools in diagnosis and healing. Besides, the book was not being written for researchers, but for patients and their physicians. The stories were picked to illustrate the science in the abutting chapters and translate it to real life.

It was impossible not to be impressed by the sense of urgency those patients conveyed, often struggling through tears, that the stories be heard and taken seriously. This may seem quite natural, considering the high drama in a typical case history; most entailed some degree of pain and struggle, and many of these patients had been trapped for years in the cycle of hope and crushing failure that typically attends the use of conventional protocols before they discovered Dr. Brown and antibiotic therapy. Each of these patients knew Dr. Brown had fought a long, solitary battle on their behalf, and there's no doubt that a lot of the emotion was related to their loyalty and gratitude for what he had endured, and the hope that he would find recognition within his lifetime.

But it also became apparent that the urgency owed to something far deeper. No one who has suffered for any length of time from inflammatory arthritis is ever free of fear that someday it could return. Every one of these patients knew their champion was old and sick, and that they were about to lose the single source of real relief many of them had ever found. Unless this book succeeded in passing his baton to other hands, in vindicating the infectious theory, and legitimizing the use of antibiotic therapy, they would be unable to receive that treatment from anyone else and could possibly find themselves back where they had started.

I managed to maintain a reasonable degree of detachment throughout the writing by consciously resisting the temptation to get caught up in those same emotions, but once the book was done I decided the infectious theory was contagious and I stopped fighting it. Tom asked me if I would be willing to serve on the steering committee of the Arthritis Institute, and I accepted without a moment's hesitation. A few months later I became a trustee.

Meanwhile, more people learned of the book as it moved nearer to publication, and on April 14, 1988, a month before its scheduled release, the first major salvo was fired in the counter-offensive against it. Dr. Paulding Phelps, then president of the American Rheumatism Association, sent a letter and "fact sheet" to every ARA member but one: Thomas McPherson Brown, a founder of the Association.

The ARA package warned that *The Road Back* was on press and beginning to receive media attention. It acknowledged the possible role of infection in causing rheumatoid arthritis, but then proceeded to attach both antibiotic therapy and Tom Brown's thesis that one infectious agent might be mycoplasmas. Phelps said, "A Special Task Force appointed by the National Institutes of Health and the National Arthritis Advisory Board did not find any sound evidence for a relationship between infection with mycoplasma and the development of rheumatoid arthritis."

It would be easy enough for a reader of that letter to infer that the "Special Task Force" had been formed to deal with the threat of pending publication of the book, but in fact there was no connection whatever. The so-called Task Force had been formed and disbanded five years earlier, its sole function having been to provide a largely cosmetic response to a request by Congress for a report on "the state of the art" of antimycoplasma treatment programs. The most recent research it discussed was the seriously flawed and widely discredited study conducted in Boston in 1971.

Two weeks later, ABC's "20/20" aired a generally depressing segment on the book based on interviews with Dr. Brown, several of his patients, and a number of establishment rheumatologists, including a new spokesman for the ARA. We sought out the opportunity to be on the show knowing there was an element of obvious risk, and even though we were disappointed with the balance between negative and positive perspectives, there was some solace in the fact that the criticism was focused almost exclusively on the fact that the theory and treatment were still unproven, and not on whether they were clinically valid.

Among Tom Brown's patients, supporters and friends who had turned on their television sets to witness the long-awaited final vindication of their hero and of the treatment that had saved many of their lives, the show was a heartbreaking disappointment. However, in response to a subsequent letter from one of those viewers, host Hugh Downs later wrote, "If the scientific community can be won over through the kinds of testing it seems to require, and the results are as Dr. Brown and his patients believe they would be, it would certainly be worth another report, but nothing in '20/20''s April 29 report was designed to attack Dr. Brown."

Apparently more neutral viewers agreed with Downs; some 15,000 copies of the book were sold in the following two weeks.

Even more telling was the response from physicians: eventually over a thousand of them would write from all over the world, requesting clinical details on the treatment protocol described in the book.

A month after "20/20," Tom was scheduled for the interview on "Good Morning America," and knowing he was seriously ill, the day before the show I flew down to New York to keep him company. We met at an apartment on Central Park, and shortly after he arrived Tom got word that a patient was trying to get in touch with him. We both knew the caller: she had been monitoring the activities of the National Institutes of Health and lobbying Congress in support of research on the infectious theory, and the message said that she had some information Tom might find useful the following morning.

Tom called the patient's home in Arizona. She said she had just learned of two unpublished experiments at the NIH's National Institute of Arthritis and Musculoskeletal and Skin Disease, and she wanted him to know about them before he went on the air. In the first, an NIH research team had succeeded in immunizing two chimpanzees against a common form of pneumonia experimentally by inducing the disease in them through oral inoculation with *Mycoplasma pneumoniae*. In the second, these same researchers and others used another form of mycoplasma, this time taken from the arthritic wrist of a human patient, and injected it into the knee of a chimpanzee. The injection induced arthritis. Just to be sure, they repeated the experiment with two more chimps and got the same result. Subsequent tests of the joint fluids from the human patient and from all three animals disclosed antibodies specific to *Mycoplasma hominis*, and the form of arthritis induced in the apes "was remarkably similar to disease in the patient."

I was on an extension phone across the room when she told us the news, and like her I was beside myself with excitement. This was the same organism Tom Brown, as a young researcher at the Rockefeller Institute, had isolated almost exactly a half-century before as a probable cause of inflammatory arthritis, and that Albert Sabin had injected into his laboratory mouse.

Instead of covering him with honor, the discovery had isolated Tom Brown as well, eventually producing a campaign of scorn and rejection that would continue to haunt him for the rest of his life. I turned to catch the expression on his face, expecting to see delight. What I saw instead was the smallest of smiles and a look of sad puzzlement.

On April 17, 1989, Thomas McPherson Brown died at the National Hospital in Arlington, Virginia, of kidney failure related to metastatic cancer. A memorial was held at the Friends Meeting House, the church he and his wife, Olive, had attended for many years when he taught at nearby George Washington University.

In the Quaker tradition, those participants who felt themselves called to say something about him stood up to speak. There were lots of people there, and nearly all of them had something to say. It was a good exercise, and the symbolism was especially appropriate to the occasion; more than one pointed out that Tom Brown had spent his life standing up, and it doesn't hurt us to do the same thing for a minute or two to say good-bye to him—or to stay on our feet when the time came for any of us to explain to others what Tom Brown had left behind.

Tom's obituary appeared in newspapers around the country. In most of them, the only quote was from someone named Connie Rabb, described as a spokeswoman for the National Institute of Arthritis and Musculoskeletal and Skin Disease of the National Instututes of Health. "Most experts by far agree that it hasn't been proven that antibiotics are an effective treatment of rheumatoid arthritis."

Just a few days after the memorial service, I had a call from Dr. Douglas Ubelaker, the curator of anthropology whom I had met at the National Museum of Natural History. He told me that a rheumatologist in Ohio had finally accomplished what Tom Brown had hoped to find in sending me to the Smithsonian two years before: Dr. Bruce M. Rothschild, director of the Arthritis Center of the Northeast Ohio University College of Medicine, had broken the code that allowed researchers to distinguish between normal postmortem erosion and the evidence of rheumatoid arthritis.

On June 5, an article titled "Tracking Rheumatoid Arthritis's Origins" described Dr. Rothschild's work in the Technology & Health section of the *Wall Street Journal.* It said he had traced the disease back some 6,500 years, that it had originated among the indigenous populations of North America, and that parallel studies produced no evidence that it reached Europe until the eighteenth century. The article also quoted the director of rheumatology at Brown University Medical School: "The origin of the disease may give us evidence about its epidemiology."

Although the cause of the disease and the means of transmission remained unknown, at the very least Rothschild's work appeared to provide new support for an infectious etiology.

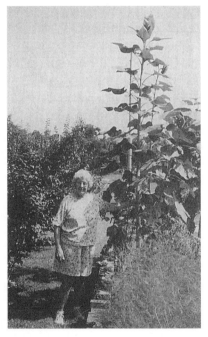

Eddie Lee Watts, eighty-one, of Ringgold, Ga., (shown in her garden with an eleven-foot sunflower), was diagnosed with rheumatoid arthritis in 1961. She also had acute undulant fever. Dr. Brown, then chief of medicine at George Washington Hospital in D.C., treated her with a combination of antibiotics.

After a year or so I began to feel like my old self, but I continued to be careful and I took my medicine religiously. Over the years, the results of this treatment have been significant.

I still take one antibiotic, one Tylenol and one vitamin E each day. I do my own work and mow my yard with both riding and push mowers. I have a garden, can and freeze foods, and am active in church and community affairs. My only deformities are two crooked big toes and a slight crook in one thumb. I told Dr. Brown he saved my life. I believe he did.

CHAPTER 4.

Testing the Infectious Theory

D r. Bruce Rothschild's thesis that rheumatoid arthritis is a communicable disease and that it originated in North America won quick and widespread acceptance in the field of anthropology. He had based his conclusions on the examination of skeletal remains from forty archeological sites from Florida through the central and eastern part of the United States all the way up to Ontario, and he had no difficulty explaining and defending his scientific technique. In medicine, too, many of his colleagues in rheumatology clearly saw what he was trying to express and were very positive and supportive. Predictably, however, there were others who were not.

Those physicians who decided to react negatively were in two camps, and their arguments would have come as no surprise to either Thomas McPherson Brown or Ignaz Phillip Semmelweis. One group said that it is necessary to have an intelligent, communicating patient who is willing to donate body fluids before it is possible to make an intelligent diagnosis, an argument that rules out learning anything from the dead along with a significant portion of the living. The other said it was not possible to differentiate between one form of inflammatory arthritis and another.

The group that raised the latter objection had been working principally on English collections of remains, and in England there is a fair amount of spondyloarthropathy, or arthritis of the spine. Spondyloarthropathy is just as inflammatory as any other rheumatoid form of the disease, and Tom Brown would have considered any such distinctions to be largely irrelevant. But they were important to Dr. Rothschild, who believed that the probable infectious cause of each form of the disease can vary widely, and that the key to eventual treatment may depend on understanding the characteristics and mechanism of each form.

LUMPERS, SPLITTERS, AND THE SEARCH FOR A TESTABLE HYPOTHESIS

For Dr. Rothschild, one of the principal motives behind his anthropological work was to carry an infectious theory about arthritis to a testable hypothesis. A few years earlier he had published on a vascular aspect of the etiology of the disease, indicating that one of the possible pathways to vascular change is an infectious agent or an allergen, and he also looked at gorillas. When he read of Tom Brown's original work at the National Zoo, he began to suspect that the disease involved in the gorilla model Tom cited was not rheumatoid arthritis as it is usually defined, but fell into the spondyloarthropathy group, specifically reactive arthritis or Reiter's syndrome. Rothschild examined the skeletons of ninety-nine gorillas that had been taken in the wild; twenty of them had a pattern of arthritis that was indistinguishable from one particular human variety of spondyloarthropathy, that associated with psoriasis.

The naturalist Dian Fossey, later to be memorialized in the film *Gorillas in the Mist*, told him that in the wild the animals often had rashes that to her looked like psoriasis. Even when physicians look at rashes, if they're not dermatologists, the reliability of diagnosis is not very good. Moreover, Rothschild knew there had been a study of cats that showed they can be subject to a rash that immunologically looks like psoriasis when the skin is examined under a microscope—and cats can indeed develop spondyloarthropathy.

To Thomas McPherson Brown, the distinctions between one form of inflammatory arthritis and another may have been meaningful in making a diagnosis, but for the most part he had observed that they seemed to respond fairly uniformly to his antibiotic therapy and so had decided they were of no particular significance to treatment. In that respect, although there were long periods in his career when that view placed him in a very small minority, he was never completely alone; there has always been a fundamental difference in views as to what comprises rheumatoid arthritis. "You put two rheumatologists in a room and you'll get three opinions," Dr. Rothschild said of the durable controversy.

The heart of the debate is that there is only a handful of major inflammatory, erosive forms of arthritis that involve more than one joint. The most common of these are rheumatoid arthritis and the spondyloarthropathy group. Diagnosticians have divided on that issue into either lumpers or splitters. Lumpers tend to group people with inflammatory arthritis together; splitters tend to separate them by characteristics. Rothschild acknowledged that the jury was still out on the question of which approach is more appropriate, although for purposes of his etiological research he had clearly sided with the splitters. Tom Brown was a lumper.

To Rothschild the distinction was more than an academic one. If the data on the patients who were being studied in the NIH-sponsored clinical trials were to be redistributed by a splitter as having one disease or the other, he had a strong hunch that the spondyloarthropathy group would be found to respond more dramatically to tetracycline. The frequency of spondyloarthropathy, based on this splitting, is as common as rheumatoid arthritis, and if Rothschild's forecast proved to be accurate, then the debate between lumping and splitting would become an extremely important issue.

Proponents of the infectious theory are aware that even the portion called rheumatoid arthritis by the narrower definition may have more than one cause. Despite that probability, when a rheumatologist looks at a person with that form of the disease anywhere in the world, the pattern of involvement is inevitably similar. By contrast, with spondyloarthropathy there is considerable variation in the way the disease presents, and in that form the variation may be a clue to causative organisms.

Rothschild was aware of Tom Brown's theory that one such agent is mycoplasma, but they are so commonplace in healthy people as well as those with rheumatoid arthritis, it is difficult to prove a causative relationship. However, he acknowledged the possibility that there's something connected to the immune system that allows these ubiquitous agents to become triggers, even though they're in everybody and most people don't get the disease. An example of the reactive arthritis phenomenon, clearly genetic in origin, turned up as an accidental by-product of a study related to diarrhea.

For the population as a whole, the frequency of one form of spondyloarthropathy is ordinarily one fourth of one percent. But the diarrhea study showed that for people with certain genes, that frequency proved to be one in four, or one hundred times higher. This revelation not only demonstrates that there are susceptibility factors, it suggests those factors may relate to which organism gets the process started. In that particular variety of arthritis, there are a half dozen organisms that can be responsible, and scientists have not yet broken down their patterns of involvement for a clue to which one may be the villain.

As dramatic as Rothschild's findings have been for those who believed them, the gradual acceptance in the medical community of rheumatoid arthritis as infectious had evolved independently of Rothschild's work on the historical etiology of the disease. By the mid-1990s, there also was no longer any question that it is transmissible—although how it's transmitted was still very much at issue. Research didn't show it as passing between spouses or in families in a direct manner. On the other hand, there are some other types of diseases, such as barley blight, that involve at least a two-component vector system, and Rothschild suspected inflammatory arthritis was probably among them. That meant two things have to happen at once before the disease could be passed along.

The trigger involved in that transmission has to be either a microorganism or an allergen. Most researchers are cautious in speculating on which specific agent it might be. Rothschild suspected it was a slow-acting agent, but he knew that when researchers looked at such diseases as Lyme arthritis, which is not caused by a slow agent, there were obvious similarities. The mystery was deepened by variations in rate of occurrence and uncertainties about the speed of onset after contact. If it really was a slow agent, the mobility of modern society virtually assured that the enigma would not be unraveled solely from an examination of present-day populations but from antiquity. The causative agent was still hidden among those things, known and unknown, which were common to the sites where it occurred in the far past. The fact that the disease preceded agriculture eliminated a whole series of possibilities and helped narrow the focus of the search.

By the time of the MIRA trials, Rothschild's research had already convinced him of the need to be much more aggressive in therapy, both by starting earlier and by using stronger suppressive agents. Despite that research, and despite his conclusion that inflammation of the joints is always erosive even if it doesn't show up immediately on X rays, those stronger agents did not yet include antibiotics. Like many other physicians, Dr. Rothschild was conscious of the issue of liability, and he described himself as a big believer that things should be done under a protocol. But he said he was very pleased that this particular protocol was finally being put to the test.

Liability was never an issue that worried Tom Brown. In the last thirty years of his practice he treated somewhere around ten thousand patients with antibiotics, and he'd never been sued by anyone. That said something about the treatment, but

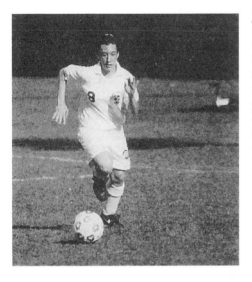

Jessie Dutton of Pottsville, Penn., was diagnosed with juvenile rheumatoid arthritis and scleroderma in the summer of 1993, at the age of twelve. A member of her school's basketball and track teams, she also played the flute and piano, and rode show horses when the two diseases literally knocked her off her feet; she was so crippled by their onset, she had to be carried in to see the doctor. Her mother recalls:

Luckily, we found Dr. Fred Burton, who had studied with Dr. Brown, in Allentown, only an hour from our home; he administered the antibiotic intravenously, and we took care of the oral form at home. By Christmas, Jessie was walking normally, gaining back her weight and getting stronger. A year later she was running again, and by the 9th grade she played varsity soccer, was one of the fastest members of the soccer team, and was back on her horse. We know that isn't the way these stories usually end, and Jessie is grateful to God for everything the experience has taught her: patience in pain, hope in struggles, and trust when there seems no way out.

it also said something about Tom Brown. Medicine is based first and foremost on personal relationships. The people who get sued the least are the ones who most nearly fulfill the image and role of the family doctor, who treat their patients as individuals and who are themselves seen as human beings by their patients.

CHAPTER 5

Witness:
Diane Aronson

The executive director of a national public interest group headquartered near Boston, Diane Aronson, fifty, looks five years younger than her age. Tall, dark-haired, healthy-looking, and pretty, she works hard at staying in shape; she works out with aerobics, she's careful of what she eats, and she keeps up her vitamins. Clearly it works.

She laughs easily and speaks in a soft but earnest voice that still hints of her childhood in Watertown, a suburb of Boston. Her youthful appearance masks more than just her true age: except for some subtle evidence of long-healed surgery on her neck, there are no visible clues to her grueling medical history.

It is unlikely that any such clues would emerge from a close examination of her childhood and early teens. Her father was executive director of the Cambridge YMCA and her mother was an officer in a bank. She was the only daughter in the family; her two older brothers were twins. She grew up tall, straight-limbed, happy, a good student. Most of all, like the rest of her family, she was healthy.

The picture, or at least the reality within that picture, began to change when she approached her late teens. It wasn't just

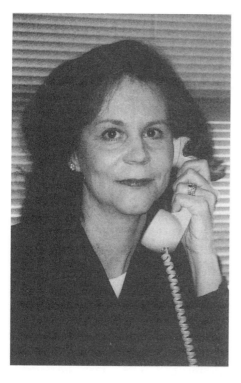

Diane Aronson, Arlington Mass., was diagnosed with RA in 1975, but her disease may have started as an undetected juvenile form a decade earlier. One of Dr. Brown's last patients, the story of her road back from terrible pain, fatigue, and near-total incapacity to a healthy, productive life comprises chapter 5 of this book. Diane is now executive director of a public-interest advocacy group in Boston.

having to have her appendix removed while she was in high school; she began to have to see physicians often for other maladies as well. She had mononucleosis in college. She developed lumps in her breasts; surgeons removed a cyst, then a tumor, both benign. Almost as ominous, especially in retrospect, were the smaller problems in between these landmarks. Starting in high school she had a number of minor illnesses, and her doctor found evidence of infection in her blood. On top of all these problems, she began to suffer intermittently—but for sustained periods of time—from enervating fatigue.

From a diagnostic viewpoint, a big part of those problem was her healthy appearance: no matter how poorly she felt, she always looked fine. Her family was constant in its love and support, but Diane's troubles were disguised by her natural buoyancy and positive approach to life. Like her family, doctors also tended to weigh the evidence of infection against the contradiction of her demeanor, and they always wound up telling her they didn't think it was anything to worry about. Because the smaller problems went largely untended, their effects began to accumulate beneath the deceptive exterior.

A few weeks after Diane's graduation from college in 1969 at age twenty-two, she married Carl, a young man whom she had known since high school, and started a job as a schoolteacher in the fall. She still tired easily and at times exhaustion seemed to rule her life. But over the next five years, even as the problem steadily worsened, she learned adaptive behavior that allowed her to stay ahead of the declining curve. Her secret to successful job performance was in the way she paced herself.

Fortunately, the fatigue didn't usually overtake her until the early afternoon, so most of her daily ration of energy was available for her work at school. But afterward, if she tried to vacuum the apartment, for example, she'd do a few strokes and then have to rest on her bed until the energy came back. She realized early on that, over the long term, pacing herself wouldn't solve the problem. And it was apparent that other aspects of her health were also deteriorating by a series of small erosions.

In planning their lives together, Diane and Carl had decided that she would only teach for a few more years because they wanted to start a family. But when months and then years passed and Diane was still not pregnant, the couple began to suspect a problem with infertility. Diane's gynecologist believed that the series of infections she brought home from school were normal—a hazard of her job—but that they might be contributing to the difficulty of conceiving.

The situation persisted with no sign of improvement. In her fifth and final year of teaching, Diane had strep throat five times, bronchitis, tonsillitis, and the mumps. Her doctors commented that her blood sedimentation level was high but then, as in the past, would brush it aside with some remark about her appearance. "Your sed rate's up, but that's probably because you've brought something home from school. That's what you've got to expect if you work around kids. Really, you look fine." Carl and Diane decided their chances would improve if she quit work and got out of the school germ pool.

Another obvious factor in her infertility, and one she couldn't have brought home from school, was endometriosis. The endometrium is a membrane in the uterus, and the condition involves the spontaneous growth of uterine cells at other sites than within the reproductive system. Although benign, this proliferation of misplaced tissue can be extremely painful. Diane suffered repeated attacks and underwent surgery several times at the end of her teaching career. The problem culminated in August of 1975 in a laparotomy, an extensive abdominal procedure that attempted to clear it up for good. It apparently worked. The next month, in September, she finally managed to conceive.

The pregnancy was the answer to the couple's prayers, but it was also to mark the opening of a new chapter in the history of Diane's health. Early in the second trimester her gynecologist noted the old problem with her blood sedimentation rate, then at 110, and referred her back to her family doctor. The internist read the other physician's report, said he, too, was concerned, and asked how she felt.

"Better than before I was pregnant," she answered. "I'm not as achy, and the fatigue isn't as bad."

He ordered more blood tests, and a few days later she received a letter. He was happy to inform her that he had diagnosed her problem: although he had initially suspected lupus, all she had was a little rheumatoid arthritis. Diane assumed from the cheerful tone that there was nothing to worry about, so she gratefully returned her attention to the concerns of her obstetrician. The pregnancy was not going as well as expected.

That physician told Diane that the rate of fetal development appeared to be abnormally slow, and he asked if she could have been a month off in estimating the date of conception. Ordinarily, it would have been easy enough to go along with such a possibility, but Diane had been keeping precise records and was sure of the conception date. He became more concerned, ordering additional tests of blood and urine and then an X ray of the fetus in utero, which Diane recognized as a sign that he suspected a serious problem.

The Aronson's daughter, Rachal, was born by Cesarean section in the spring of 1976. She was a frail baby, weighing only 5 pounds 7 ounces, and despite her mother's constant attention would fuss or cry loudly for what seemed like hours at a time. One day, when the infant was still only a few months old, Diane noticed with alarm that Rachal was starting to become cyanotic. She immediately called the pediatrician and told him that her daughter was turning blue.

The doctor explained that Rachal's condition indicated insufficient oxygen in the blood. The infant was hospitalized the following day, but it would be almost three years before anyone could provide a reasonable explanation for the cause of the malady. Meanwhile, the problem was compounded with severe digestive malabsorption, and Rachal's little stomach became bloated like those of starving children in Ethiopia and Somalia. For a brief time Rachal was diagnosed as having seizures and put on anticonvulsant medication, to which she reacted terribly. Eventually, after many trips to the hospital and countless examinations of her heart, the problem was found instead to be a vasomotor disorder resulting from her premature birth, and she outgrew it.

Catastrophes seldom come by halves. Shortly after the birth and even before the infant's medical problems, Diane suffered the first major flare-up of her arthritis. On top of which she developed a breast infection while nursing Rachal. The doctors were reluctant to medicate either condition for fear of contaminating the baby, but decided to treat the breast infection anyway because otherwise the nursing would have to be stopped. Fortunately, Rachal showed no reaction to the antibiotic.

Almost immediately afterward, however, Rachal's behavior became violently erratic without any apparent cause. Many months later, when she was switched to solid foods, doctors realized Rachal was allergic to some of the foods Diane had been eating that were then passed along in her milk to the infant. Rachal spent much of her days and nights screaming in rage or agony. Between Diane's own pain, depression, and fatigue from the untreated arthritis and the continually rising demands for attention from a newborn whose survival was in serious doubt, the new mother began each day with dread and ended it in complete physical and emotional exhaustion.

Several months later, when baby Rachal was no longer directly dependent on her mother for nourishment, Diane's internist started her on medication to try dealing with the arthritis. The treatment followed a classic path. He began with a liquid form of aspirin, then successively moved her to Motrin, Feldene, and finally Clinoril. All of them had side effects, and as Diane went from one drug to the next, the side effects became progressively more harmful. She suffered from extremely painful colitis, and eventually wound up in the emergency room at her local hospital with blood in her stool. The internist didn't appear particularly surprised, and although he was sympathetic he assured her the reaction was nothing to worry about: she should expect that these things might happen from time to time. No reference was made to her medication.

It would be more than another decade before medical scientists reported that the same "mild" medicines Diane was taking for her arthritis were responsible for killing up to 30,000 people every year with silent ulcers. Certainly it was never suggested to her that she might die.

Some months later, the same doctor who diagnosed Diane's arthritis found a malignant melanoma in her neck. In retrospect, there is no doubt that the discovery saved her life. By the time he spotted it, however, the cancer was well into Level Two and required radical surgery that almost cost her an ear. Because of the severity of the procedure, large skin grafts were taken from Diane's leg and she left the hospital on crutches in even greater pain. In the following decade, five corrective operations had to be performed.

During those long, dark months, Diane would look at the beautiful child—for whose life she had waited so long and patiently—and wonder how she could possibly take care of her. And she wondered if she would be around for Rachal as she grew up. It was a sad, scary time.

Somehow they both managed to survive. Over the following years, a day at a time, their health stabilized, and the child's even began to improve. By the time Rachal was ten or eleven, there was evidence she was outgrowing all the problems of her infancy and early childhood. She did well in school and developed a real talent as a classical pianist. The pained and frightened baby was turning into a happy, well-adjusted young lady, a parent's dream.

Diane's own recovery from cancer was slower and less dramatic, but with each passing year it seemed more and more likely that the operation had indeed saved her life. In the meantime—although she had ups and downs—she managed, by guarding carefully against exhaustion and by being extremely careful of her diet, to keep her arthritis under tenuous control, with a minimum of medication.

Despite occasional flare-ups and persistent stomach problems, she even went back to work. She became executive director of a peace-advocacy program. During her tenure the membership grew from less than a hundred to 25,000, and eventually she co-chaired a coalition of like-minded organizations with a combined constituency of over three million. Diane was equally successful in her home life and found she was able to do almost all of the things as a mother that she had once feared would be denied her. In the spring of 1987 she decided to leave her job, partly with the intention of spending more time with her family.

Then, out of the blue, she experienced the worst rheumatic flareup of her life. Her feet felt like cement blocks, and the pain was so intense the only way she could move across a room was a tortuous step at a time. The most trivial demands of housework and parenting became monumental challenges. She couldn't go shopping with Rachal, and even waddling from one room to another within her own home caused tears of pain and desperation to stream down her face.

Almost as frightful as her physical agony was the knowledge that she was now facing the next plateau in medication. In the early stages of her affliction Diane had studied the progression of debilitating side effects that arrived with each new step in her arthritis treatment from supposedly mild drugs; and now she felt helpless, as if she were being pulled down into the deep end of a dark and frightening abyss.

One Friday night in late April, just a few weeks after the flare-up that had so completely undone her life, a friend called to tell Diane to turn on the television program "20/20"; it was about a doctor in a hospital just outside Washington who had written a book on antibiotic therapy as a promising alternative treatment for rheumatoid arthritis.

The title of the segment, "Selling False Hope?" was clearly intended to suggest a fair degree of skepticism, and Diane didn't expect to be at all encouraged by what was to come. Despite the negative tone of the promotional bites, however, the segment itself left her more confused and curious than convinced. The minute the show ended, the friend called and asked her, "What do you think?" Diane answered that she didn't know. They talked for a few minutes, and Diane finally agreed she'd try to get a copy of the book mentioned on the program and judge its merits for herself.

Two weeks later, Carl and Diane left for a long-planned birthday weekend of rest and inactivity at a quaint old country inn called the Wooden Goose in Cape Neddick, Maine. The drive was difficult, but by then Diane had picked up a copy of *The Road Back*, and once in their room she stretched herself out painstakingly on the bed and read the book from cover to cover. She was amazed at how accurately the patients' histories described the symptoms of her disease, and how lucidly Dr. Brown explained their meaning. When a passage described a familiar phenomenon or feeling that she had been unable to articulate herself, she would read it aloud to Carl. The book gave them their first real understanding of how arthritis worked, and it gave her a strong, fresh sense that there was reason to hope. Perhaps equally important, it gave them new insight into the role of depression in Diane's illness.

Everyone knows that in life reason and emotions don't always work hand-in-hand—and this is especially true when that life has been filled with illness. But from mid-adolescence Diane had often found it difficult to control her feelings of sadness, and some of her most difficult teenage memories were of occasions in which tears got the better of her. The feelings of despair had become far more profound since her first arthritic flare-up. They were so bad that she finally mentioned them to her rheumatologist. The doctor listed with great sympathy and referred her to a psychiatrist. There was never any suggestion by either physician that the depression was a part of the arthritis.

On the contrary, until their holiday at the Wooden Goose, she and Carl had both simply accepted this frailty as the product of her basic temperament, albeit exacerbated by disease and exhaustion. On reading the book, they discovered to their amazement that it was an absolutely normal clinical symptom of her physical condition, as much a part of rheumatoid arthritis as the pain and weakness. Her real temperament, they realized, was the optimistic, cheerful, strong personality that had helped create and build a national organization, that had risen above the cancer and struggled with the arthritis, allowing her to lead a useful, fulfilling life as a wife and mother.

Diane had enough experience in problem solving and in business that she didn't just throw down the book and rush right out to claim the new messiah. She set about to systematically gather more data, starting with a call the following Monday to the Arthritis Institute where Tom Brown practiced. She was told that he was booked solid for the next nine months, but considering the popularity of the book that was pretty much what she expected. All right, she said, how could she get in touch with some of his patients?

That evening Diane spoke with a woman in Virginia named Myra Frank. Myra confirmed her experience as set out in *The Road Back* and referred Diane to another patient, in the Boston area, named Jane Fagan. Over the course of the next several days the chain of referrals crossed the country, and each time Diane spoke with a new voice on the telephone it told her of a case history that had many of the same landmarks as her own. Slowly, as the evidence continued to accumulate, she became more and more optimistic that this relatively risk-free treatment might work for her as well.

Nearer to home, however, not everyone she spoke with proved to be true believers in the infectious theory and antibiotic therapy. Her new rheumatologist had told Diane that her rheumatoid factor, which is a measurement of the disease that physicians view with alarm when it approaches 75 or 100, had gone off the charts at 10,000. A few days after reading the book, Diane was in Boston for a checkup and asked her new doctor what he thought of Dr. Brown. The physician rummaged in his desk and produced the letter from the American Rheumatism Association. He read parts of it to her and dismissed the subject with two words: "Pure quackery."

That summer, on a referral from Tom Brown's appointments nurse, Diane interviewed Dr. John Sinnott in Ida Grove, Iowa, and a few days later flew out with her mother and began receiving the antibiotic therapy described in the book.

It proved to be an astonishing experience. Diane had never been to Iowa before. Ida Grove was a town of only 2,000, and the hospital where Dr. Sinnott practiced was a small, neat building next to a cornfield. Despite the hope with which she undertook the adventure, as the days passed and the treatment continued (Dr. Sinnott felt her symptoms were serious enough that he administered the antibiotic intravenously) there were times when the feelings of depression were irresistible. Sinnott had a gentle, reassuring manner and he reaffirmed that those dark dips in mood came with the territory. But even through the tears, Diane noticed something else.

For most of her life she had suffered from infected sinuses— a problem so acute that she could peel onions without even smelling them. But she and her mother were out for a ride along the country roads one afternoon after her daily session at the clinic, and suddenly Diane could smell fresh tobacco smoke. She looked around for the source, but at first all she could see was a nearly empty highway between endless fields of ripening corn. Then she noticed that far ahead of them was a farmer's pick-up. She asked her mother to increase their speed. A minute later, when they overtook the truck, Diane had her first view of the man at the wheel—and she saw that he was smoking a large cigar.

She looked at her mother in amazement. As they continued the drive, she realized she could smell the country air, and the odors of flowers, of ripening corn, of green grass, were more vivid than any other during the past decade. After just a few days of antibiotic therapy, the sinus problem had quietly gone into remission. Something was happening.

That wasn't the only sign. Diane's turbulent medical history included severe stomach problems—a recent endoscopic examination had confirmed both gastritis and esophagitis—and she consumed large quantities of gastric medicine containing calcium. She discussed with Dr. Sinnott the fact that calcium could interfere with the absorption of the antibiotic and agreed to try to get through the therapy without using them or any other medicines. She did, and to her amazement she never needed them again. The stomach problems seemed to have disappeared along with the sinus infection.

Four years later Diane would think back to that unexplained remission when she learned of work performed by a team of medical researchers in Texas. Dr. David Y. Graham, a gastroenterologist at the Veterans' Affairs Medical Center in Houston, reported in the May 1992 issue of *Annals of Internal Medicine* that his team's research provided "compelling evidence . . . that peptic ulcer . . . is the end result of a bacterial infection." That meant that peptic ulcers had little or nothing to do with heredity or the lifestyle choices such as tobacco, stress, and alcohol on which they traditionally had been blamed. The paper went on to say that those disorders, both of which are symptomatically identical to the problems that so long afflicted Diane Aronson, can be cured 100 percent of the time by a safe, easy, inexpensive combination of Tagamet and tetracycline.

But if the sinus and stomach problems both seemed headed for remission by the time Diane returned home from Ida Grove, the disease she had gone there to cure appeared to have settled in with a vengeance. She sat in the dining room of her hillside home in Arlington, Massachusetts, crying bitterly, and told Carl and Rachal she didn't know how she could live through the pain. She could barely move. The depression was blacker and deeper than at any time in her life, and the fatigue was so immense that she could barely stay awake even with her weeping.

If there was one thing that kept her going and that helped her stick with the medication, it was the knowledge from the book and from her conversation with Dr. Sinnott of what was really taking place within her body. She recognized that she was suffering from the Herxheimer reaction, which meant the medication was working. Three months after she began the therapy in Iowa, Diane noticed that the symptoms had begun to slowly dissipate, and that she was getting better.

It was noticeable in the little things. The tears were less frequent. Her stamina began to slowly return, and she was able to get through whole days without the pathological need for sleep. She could walk across the room, even up and down the stairs, without the terrible pain. Some days were better than others, but in this slow accrual of small blessings she recognized a new pattern that was forming in her life.

The following January, partly through Jane Fagan's advocacy on her behalf, Diane was finally offered an appointment with Dr. Brown, and because Washington was so much nearer than Iowa, she quickly accepted. There were other reasons as well, of course. She knew from Jane that Dr. Brown was nearing the end of his life, and she leapt at the chance to meet the physician whose work and study—and, above all, persistence in the face of every kind of opposition—had so dramatically reordered her own future. During the same trip, Jane invited her, with Dr. Brown's blessing, to join a newly formed steering committee of the Arthritis Institute. Eager to return a part of what she had been given, she accepted that as well. Diane also realized, despite the improvements that continued to accumulate following her therapy with Dr. Sinnott, that her own odyssey with arthritis was far from over. She was still subject to occasional, if less frequent, flare-ups and all that went with them. Her own road back promised to be a long one.

The morning they met, Dr. Brown's physician's assistant warned Diane that he was having a poor day and that the staff had been trying unsuccessfully to convince him to go home. The assistant sat with them through the interview, which started off with Tom's typical warmth and interest in his patient. But the energy level didn't last; three times between Diane's answer to his questions about her personal history, it was apparent from his eyes and the hesitancy of his response that he was wavering on unconsciousness. Diane fought against the lump she felt forming in her throat, and was relieved for him when the meeting came to an end and the physician's assistant led her across the hall to the room where she would be given her IV.

I met Diane Aronson for the first time on the evening of that same day. Like her, Jane Fagan and I had flown down for the initial session of the new steering committee, and our group convened in a conference room at the National Hospital. In the course of a short conversation among the three Bostonians on the committee after the meeting broke up, Diane asked me if I could suggest a physician closer to home who might be persuaded to follow her antibiotic treatment. She was already greatly improved, but she knew that she had a long way still to go. Her journey would be a lot easier if she had someone near at hand to monitor the treatment, to check her sed rate, liver function, and rheumatoid factor, and perhaps to even help her over the occasional hurdles.

It was less than a year since the book had appeared, and instead of lowering resistance to Tom Brown's theory and treatment, the publicity that had followed its publication seemed to have caused it to intensify. Diane's experience with her rheumatologist was hardly unique, but one could only guess at how

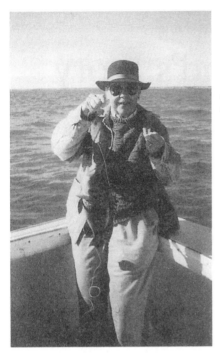

Jean Jones, rheumatoid arthritis, Cape Cod, Mass.

In 1991, I became a test subject for the MIRA research project. What did I have to lose? I was almost 60 years old and had suffered from this disease ever since being diagnosed with juvenile RA as a little girl. Both hips and both knee joints had been replaced, my shoulder joints were frozen, and my elbows had lost their full range of motion. Although I discovered after the study that I was in the placebo group, in 1994 I started taking the same minocycline therapy that had been proven safe and effective to so many others in the study. Six months later my rheumatoid factor was negative, there were no signs of inflammation, and I was in remission.

many thousands of prospective patients had been deterred from getting help by other doctors reading them that letter from the American Rheumatism Association.

After thinking about it for a while, I told her I didn't know where it might lead, but that she might get in touch with David Trentham at Beth Israel Hospital.

CHAPTER 6

A Husband's Story

Years ago, when the doctor finally eliminated the other possibilities and diagnosed Diane's arthritis, Carl Aronson didn't have any idea what to expect. He recalled hearing his parents and others in their generation when they complained about aching and stiffness in their joints, but their tone had always been stoical and accepting, similar to when they spoke about bad weather, or fatigue from hard work, or simply the problems everyone had to expect from growing old. Whatever was going on with his wife was different in degree, but some months would pass before he came to fully appreciate that it was also different in kind.

The doctor's comment on Diane's pregnancy offered an ominous early signal of the seriousness of the disease. "You'd better plan to put all your eggs in one basket," he told them. "One child is about all you'll be able to handle."

Carl was as shocked as Diane. As bad as her illness had been up to that point, neither of them had the sense that it was anything that couldn't eventually be fixed, or that there were any serious long-term limits on their lives. Now, despite what had seemed almost cavalier casualness toward her diagnosis, the doctor clearly had a different view of what lay ahead. Far from looking forward to improvement, he seemed to be pointing to a long, arduous, downhill journey for them both.

Shortly after the diagnosis, they recalled another model in their lives for what it meant to have arthritis. A year or two before Diane's pregnancy, the young couple had made a vacation trip to Venezuela. On a cable car climbing a mountainside, they struck up an acquaintance with a fellow tourist, an American woman in her fifties from New York. The woman had difficulty getting out of her seat at the end of the ride, and Carl had helped her up. Her arms, they both noticed, were terribly frail and crippled, and she was obviously in great pain when she tried to walk. The Aronsons spent a fair amount of time with her through the rest of their trip and stayed in touch by telephone and letter on their return to Boston. Now, looking back on that episode with different eyes, they realized that the woman might well have been holding up a mirror to their own future, and the thought was frightening.

A few years later, Diane and Carl had a reason to visit New York, and they went to see their friend from the cable car. They found her confined to her bed, her face and joints swollen and inflamed with the disease and the drugs she had been given to combat it, so changed in appearance they hardly recognized her. She was in such pain the only position she could tolerate was lying on her side with her back to them, talking to the wall. She lived less than a year after that visit.

The deterioration of their friend was doubly shocking for its parallels with what was happening to Diane. During the early years of their marriage, a pattern had already begun that would continue through much of their daughter's childhood. Diane was so exhausted by the time she got home, she simply collapsed; dinnertime was not in the family's dining room but in her bed. By the time Rachal was in school, she told her parents she wished they could be like other families and eat occasional dinners at a table. Carl did the shopping, prepared the food, cleaned the house, and served as both his wife's home health aide and their daughter's nursemaid. The manager of the Chinese restaurant knew all three of them by their first names.

Another aspect of the disease they couldn't have foreseen was the difficulty it created in trying to schedule any kind of a social life. Plans made in the morning with the best of intentions would often fall victim by nighttime to pain, fatigue, and overwhelming depression, and Carl would find himself calling friends or business associates to beg off from their earlier commitments. It wasn't always easy to explain; Diane's disease had done little to her appearance, and to their acquaintances she was bright, beautiful, healthy, normal—if also perhaps a bit less than the life of every party.

Although Diane was the one who collected most of the information on her disease, Carl found himself in a new relationship to that information when together they both began reading *The Road Back*. For the first time, he was able to see both his wife and himself in a description of her illness, to verify her own sense of its relevance, and to share her excitement as they looked together into this new mirror that reflected their experience and, at long last, a sense of hope.

The changes the arthritis required in their lives didn't all come at once, of course, but paced the slow, erosive nature of the illness. The journey back to recovery brought adjustments as well, and although they were of a far happier kind, they had in common with the downhill leg of their trip that they were never sudden or spectacular. At the start, as Diane began to improve, she would sometimes accompany Carl when he visited the market to do their shopping. Then, after a time, she was able to do the shopping on her own, but Carl would still have to bring the bags into the house. Eventually, she reached the point where she could do it all.

"At the beginning," Carl remembers, "it was all Diane could do to channel her energy to the absolutely necessary tasks of the day, and by the time she got home from work it was almost as though I had to catch her as she collapsed. It was hard, but through it all we learned to work as partners, and that's a pretty good thing. Today she has more energy than almost any-

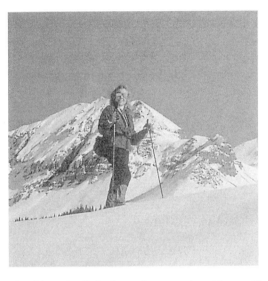

Joy Bush, Los Alamos, N.M., was diagnosed with RA in 1966.

Since then, I have had 18 surgeries on my hands and feet, including the excision of 11 joints and the replacement of a metacarpal. It wasn't until 1984 that I met Dr. Brown, and began antibiotic therapy. It was a late start and a hard battle against multiple infectious causes, but at last I'm in remission. I'm able to do all the things I want to do, with no stiffness, no pain, and greatly improved endurance. The treatment has controlled my disease.

one I know, and she makes the most of every minute. There are still times, though less and less frequent, when she has a flare, and the old fatigue and pain catch up with her for a few days at a time—but we know how to work together to deal with it. As painful as this experience has been, we're both grateful for the lessons in it. We use them every day."

CHAPTER 7

Clinical Evidence

B eth Israel Hospital in Boston is a teaching hospital of Harvard Medical School, and Dr. David Trentham, who happens to be a long-time friend and colleague of Bruce Rothschild, is head of the department of rheumatology there. A quiet, scholarly southerner, in the late 1980s Dr. Trentham was not as well known to the general public as Dr. Rothschild, as the nature of his inquiries was far less accessible to scrutiny or even understanding by the popular press than Rothschild's anthropological detective work. Within the narrower world of medical science, however, Trentham was widely recognized as one of the foremost researchers into the infectious etiology of inflammatory arthritis, and many of the most important milestones in this arcane science bear his signature.

I didn't actually contact David Trentham until shortly after publication of *The Road Back*, when someone told me about a paper, which he had delivered in Arizona, that discussed rheumatoid arthritis as an infectious disease. Like Tom Brown, he had impressive credentials: an associate professor of medicine at Harvard, the author of scores of papers, he had been an

NIH research grant recipient for over a decade, and had been the principal investigator on four separate clinical protocols for the treatment of rheumatoid arthritis. But despite the fact that he and Tom Brown were both fishing in the same water, it was hard to imagine anyplace more entrenched in the establishment than Harvard Medical School; and, furthermore, I had no way of knowing how Dr. Trentham might have been influenced by the American Rheumatism Association's campaign against Tom Brown and the book. At that point Tom's health was declining so badly that travel was out of the question, and without his aegis and no medical degree of my own I was somewhat chary about calling a prominent physician whom I had never met to discuss his work. When I finally mustered the nerve, I couldn't have been more thrilled with the result.

Far from being hostile or aloof, Dr. Trentham astonished me with his openness, understanding, and respect for the work to which Tom Brown had dedicated his life. We met a couple of times in Boston that fall and winter. Both the research director and administrator of the Arthritis Institute of the National Hospital flew to Boston to discuss mutual goals, and Dr. Trentham made a reciprocal trip to the Institute in Virginia. All of Tom Brown's patients, colleagues, and friends were painfully aware of the limits on his remaining time and Dr. Trentham's appearance on the scene came as a tremendous relief and source of hope for those who were looking for a new standard bearer to carry on Dr. Brown's tattered banner.

In early 1990, Dr. Trentham gave me a paper that had just been published in *The Journal of Rheumatology* by a Dutch physician named Ferdinand Breedveld, based on work that he had begun a couple of years earlier as one of Trentham's research associates at Beth Israel. Titled *Minocycline Treatment for Rheumatoid Arthritis: An Open Dose-Finding Study*, it reported on the experience of ten patients in the Netherlands who had taken oral minocycline (a form of tetracycline) for a period of only sixteen weeks. As such studies go, it fell far short of the requirements for proof: the test group was too small, and the time period almost laughably short, and there was no e-blind control. But there was nothing laughable about the abstract of the results:

> *Half of the efficacy variables improved significantly after four weeks of therapy. At the end of the study all variables were significantly changed compared with their pre-treatment values. We conclude that minocycline may be beneficial in RA. This effect needs to be confirmed in controlled studies.*

After reading the paper, I told Trentham of a letter Tom Brown had received from a doctor named Joseph Mercola in Schaumburg, Illinois, shortly after *The Road Back* had first appeared. Mercola had a young patient with the juvenile form of rheumatoid arthritis, and after reading the physician's protocol in the book he had begun Dr. Brown's treatment with the same form of antibiotic that would be used later in the Dutch study. Dr. Mercola's letter said he had been misled by the book's continued insistence that therapeutic results take months or even years: the little girl started to respond to treatment within the first few days, and within a matter of weeks she was completely cured. It was hardly a complaint; Mercola went on to treat hundreds of rheumatoid arthritics in the following years, becoming one of the most experienced antibiotic therapists in the country, and one of the treatment's staunchest advocates.

The year after Tom Brown died, Dr. Trentham invited me to lunch at the Harvard Club in Boston, along with a couple of patients I had sent his way in the previous months. One of them was Diane Aronson. The other was my old friend from the Caribe Playa, Jane Fagan.

At that meeting, Dr. Trentham told us of his proposal, once the NIH clinical trials were fully subscribed and under way, for establishing the Dr. Thomas McPherson Brown Professorship in Rheumatology at Harvard Medical School and Beth Israel Hospital. In turn, I told him that the publisher was planning a new edition of *The Road Back*, and I asked him if he had any suggestions for bringing the story up to date. He immediately offered to provide an overview of the advances in arthritis research which had taken place since the book originally appeared.

Because of another publishing commitment, I was unable to take him up on that offer until late the following summer. When we finally did meet again, this time in his office at Beth Israel, it was obvious that ever since Tom Brown's death the climate and direction of arthritis research had undergone dramatic change. Researchers had developed new insights into the relationship between infection and immunity. They were in the midst of a major reappraisal of the true efficacy of traditional treatments, including a hard, critical look at the relatively new

Karen Easton, Long Island, N.Y., started dancing at age two, got into ballet at twelve, and stayed with it for the next two decades until RA forced her to quit both performing and teaching in 1989. But that didn't stop the disease.

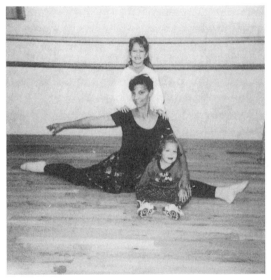

My old injuries were getting worse and not healing, and the arthritis was winning the battle. By early 1997 I had to retire to the couch daily because of joint pain, fatigue, and the overall awful feeling. I have two small children, and my options were to increase the plaquenil and prednisone—or really bite the bullet and try the minocin and pray it worked.

Seven months later I was off the other medicines entirely. I am a real active mom and take my kids to their activities and enjoy them immensely. Most amazing of all, I'm able to dance again and teach ten classes a week. In my wildest dreams, I never would imagine going from the couch to the dance studio in seven months. I'm grateful for the miracle.

therapeutic standards of the past decade. Most tellingly of all, even as the medical community organized itself for the long-awaited clinical trials of Tom Brown's antibiotic therapy, researchers had already begun to explore the intricate and surprising mechanism by which tetracycline achieved at least a part of its effects. The momentum had continued to build after Tom's death, just as we had all hoped it would. The arthritis breakthrough was at hand, and the new purpose of the interview was to examine how it was occurring.

Before we began that examination, however, Dr. Trentham wanted to speak for the record about the first edition of *The Road Back*. He considered it "very important that the new edition preserve the original text intact, first and foremost as recording of a major historic cornerstone in the treatment, and in our understanding and in our concepts, of rheumatoid arthritis." I agreed; for all the controversy it engendered just four years earlier, the book had proven to be a remarkably reliable map for much that followed, and this was the logical place to examine it again, before considering its aftermath.

Although for reasons of privacy the identity and personal story of one patient have been deleted, all the other case histories and all of Tom Brown's original insights into the mechanism and treatment of this disease are reproduced in this edition as well, exactly as they first appeared.

PART II

THE ROAD BACK

Rheumatoid Arthritis: Its Cause and Its Treatment

Thomas McPherson Brown, M.D., and Henry Scammell

To our wives, Olive and Caroline,
for their faith,

to the volunteers and staff of the Arthritis Institute,
for their support,

to Rob Maguire and Doug Reddan,
for giving the Institute its start and sustenance,

to Jane Fagan,
for everything, especially her introduction,

To Tom Hallowell,
for a lifetime of friendship
and for his financial backing when it counted most,

to all the members of Tom Brown's Army, 10,000 strong,
for their abiding courage,

and particularly to those whose stories are on these pages,
for their generosity,

this book is lovingly dedicated by the authors.

CHAPTER 8

The Road Back

A rthritis has been with the human race longer than any other known disease—perhaps since our most distant ancestors first stood upright. But unlike other scourges of the ancient past, it is still very much with us: in addition to being man's oldest affliction, it is also the most widespread, affecting one out of every seven people on the planet.

It is not a minor disorder or a simple inconvenience. Arthritis can disfigure hands, twist spines, paralyze joints, weaken the connective tissue in hearts and other vital organs, and create fatigue, intense depression, and agonizing pain. Today, over a hundred different forms of the disease collectively afflict some 37 million Americans, and that number is growing at a rate of over a million cases every year. The price, including various forms of treatment and the cost of lost productivity, has been estimated at as much as $50 billion a year, or $1 billion a week, in this country alone.

The reason these numbers remain so astronomical even in this age of advanced technology is that pharmaceutical research took a serious wrong turn just before the middle of this century, one that created a forty-year detour in the search for the cause and cure of rheumatoid arthritis. As a result of that wrong turn, the American medical establishment was left with little choice but to treat the disease as an act of God. Patients were told they were born to have the disease through heredity, or that it was produced by stress, injury, a glandular defect, or aging, and that nothing could be done to avoid it or to cure it. For many years since that time, the approach to treatment has been purely symptomatic.

A TRAGIC FAILURE

Treatment of the symptoms of rheumatoid arthritis is now one of America's major industries. Judged purely in terms of profits, it is among the most successful. Judged by results, it is a tragic failure.

Even forty years ago, it was obvious that none of these speculations on the probable mechanism of rheumatoid arthritis held water. It is true that there are families in which arthritis is endemic, but there are many other instances in which there has been only a single case in three generations, which of course confutes the hereditary concept. As to aging as a cause, one only has to consider the hundreds of thousands of victims of juvenile rheumatoid arthritis or the millions of arthritics who are still in their teens and twenties. Stress is even less substantial: most highly stressed people never get arthritis, and many people who have very little stress in their lives suddenly find themselves afflicted. Another "explanation" for the disease is that it is caused or can be cured by diet. Nearly every disease is influenced to a certain extent by what we eat, and the nutritional link to arthritis has been worked over hundreds of different ways. There is some evidence, for example, that Eskimos have less arthritis than the rest of us—but there is no clear proof that it is because they consume so much fish oil.

The effect of all this confusion was a general abrogation of responsibility for finding the real cause of the disease, and pharmaceutical companies turned their attention elsewhere;

the formulation and manufacture of arthritis pain relievers eventually would become one of the biggest businesses in the world.

Cortisone came along at about that time, and its dramatic initial impact on the inflammation and pain of rheumatoid arthritis was interpreted at first as an indication that the basic cause of the disease was a glandular deficiency. Cortisone was a natural body product, after all, and if it worked so well on arthritis, it must be that the arthritic's body wasn't producing the required amount. From there it was a short step to characterizing arthritis as an autoimmune response. This view of the disease as the body fighting its own cells was a convenient one, and this convenience soon translated into unyielding dogma.

There were three basic problems with the autoimmune theory. It was accepted before it was proven. It went against prior evidence. It was based on flawed logic. A fourth problem was that it essentially derailed all further efforts to pursue an understanding of the real cause of the disease for the next three decades.

GOING FOR THE CAUSE

As a young clinician and researcher in this field, I was aware that no major disease had ever been understood or conquered until its cause had been identified. I also knew that serendipity favors medical research only when the investigator is on the right path to begin with, and that nobody ever stumbled onto the North Pole while they were headed south. The problem of finding the right starting place in the search for the cause of rheumatoid arthritis was comparable to coming from another culture and being asked to explain the exploded atomic bomb; no doubt one of the last things one would think of is the splitting of the atom. But I was determined to find the right starting point, the one that pointed due north to the cause.

The first clue I had that the cause of rheumatoid arthritis was an infectious agent that produced a damaging type of allergic reaction came from a simple clinical observation.

I was a third-year medical student at Johns Hopkins, using my free time to work in the Arthritis Clinic; it was an area in which the patients had great needs, and little was known. Gold salts were being administered, as they are today, and almost invariably the patient became much worse following the first injection. Yet with subsequent weekly injections, most patients gradually improved. This seemed to indicate that there was a hidden causative factor that was being stirred up at the start, but with continued treatment that factor was being reduced.

At the time the rest of the arthritis research establishment embarked on this long excursion down the byway of symptomatic treatment, I took on new duties as professor and chairman of the Department of Medicine at George Washington University in Washington, D.C. I was also a member of the American Rheumatism Association Committee on Public Relations, a body whose principal function was to interpret medical dogma for the American consumer. As director of the Department of Medicine, with philosophical as well as scientific responsibilities to the students, I soon found myself compelled to take a stand against the trend, by then widespread, toward the indiscriminate use of large doses of cortisone for pain relief in arthritis.

In large doses, cortisone weakens the immune system, and simple logic tells us this can only lead to trouble; the benefits of pain relief are soon offset by serious complications associated with the reduction of the body's natural defense mechanism. We had already seen tuberculosis become activated in the presence of cortisone treatment, as well as the transformation of chicken pox and measles from mild childhood illnesses into lethal disease processes due to uncontrolled pneumonia and meningitis that developed when the immunity was weakened.

Conversely, I wasn't against the use of cortisone altogether.

Small doses had been shown to help arthritics by modifying their allergic state, allowing other medicines to become more effective. But large doses had the opposite effect, interfering with any treatment program that depended on the immune system for its support.

THE FIRST VICTIM OF CORTISONE

Ironically, it was the advent of cortisone, which was an undeniably valuable discovery, that pulled the rug out from under any attempt to go for the cause of rheumatoid arthritis. The actual event when this occurred was a meeting of the American Rheumatism Association in Atlantic City in the early 1950s. I was one of five panelists invited to discuss cortisone and its use.

At that time, cortisone was still a very expensive drug to manufacture, and the head of the arthritis program at the National Institutes of Health, a Dr. Joseph Bunim, was advocating a cortisone subsidy from Congress. He was primarily a researcher rather than a practitioner, and he disregarded the risks in favor of the drug's dramatic effect on the relief of pain. Dr. Bunim declared, as did the drug's discoverer, that cortisone for arthritis was really comparable to insulin for diabetes, and that any difficulties with the drug could be overcome with further research.

The moderator opened the panel discussion before an audience of several thousand physicians by asking me for my views in regard to the use of cortisone. I took a deep breath and said that in large doses it was an extremely dangerous drug—that it should be used sparingly if at all. My statement was equivalent to coming out against mother's milk; I knew I was stepping into the fiery furnace, but I had no choice.

Dr. Bunim didn't take it at all well. He felt that winning a consensus of this audience of doctors was essential to gain final approval for the subsidy legislation then in Congress, and my remarks could do great harm to his efforts. He stood up and said in a voice shaking with fury that my statement was totally irresponsible.

The moderator, who was from the Mayo Clinic where cortisone had been initially developed, objected to Bunim's response. He said that I had a perfect right to my views, that the Association appreciated hearing them, and that Dr. Bunim's comments were uncalled for. As Bunim settled angrily into his seat, I could see my fortunes settling with him; I knew that from that time on I would be in trouble with the Establishment. Cortisone was indeed a lethal weapon, and one of its first victims was the voice of opposition.

A number of physicians in the audience came up to the stage after the meeting and congratulated me for taking a strong stand, saying that they, too, had encountered some serious problems with the drug. But within two weeks, I received a call from an officer of the American Rheumatism Association asking politely if I would be willing to withdraw from membership on the Public Relations committee. He told me he wanted to be sure that others in the membership would have the opportunity to serve in this responsible and highly visible position. I laughed and said, "Come on, George, who are you kidding? You guys are going to be sore at me forever."

I also told him that as chairman of the Department of Medicine, I said what I did because I had a responsibility to the truth. He said my remarks about cortisone had nothing to do with it. There was no doubt where all this was going, and I had neither the time nor the inclination to pursue a course that could only end in futility and rancor, so I withdrew my name.

Shortly afterward, Congress voted to subsidize the production of cortisone.

From that time on, our funding for research into the cause of arthritis at George Washington University nearly disappeared and we had to scrounge for every penny.

The main thrust of arthritis research in America spent itself unproductively in the cul-de-sac of metabolic dysfunction and autoimmunity for the next thirty years. It is only in the past decade that it began at last to find its way back to the main road.

RETURNING TO THE MAIN ROAD

When an inexperienced hunting dog is first exposed to game, he uses all of his energy searching for tracks in an open field, running in circles, chasing after every lead regardless of how fresh or stale. A researcher in the cause of arthritis is faced with the same apparently endless number of possibilities, with the potential for at least as much frustration and hopelessness. But like the hunting dog, he eventually learns which directions are most likely to be productive and he begins to establish a set of priorities. And he starts to get results.

This book describes how the dogs that have been hunting for the infectious cause of arthritis eventually got smart, what they found, and why they are now about to become the Most Popular Breed.

It deals with all the rheumatoid forms of arthritis, which means every form except osteoarthritis. With that single exception, all the many and varied types of this affliction have an inflammatory component, they all show evidence of connective-tissue damage, and they all are under the aegis of a process which resembles the autoimmune reaction.

A real autoimmune reaction is the body fighting its own cells. In rheumatoid arthritis, the body does not attack its own cells as the primary target. What is called the autoimmune reaction in all these forms of arthritis is actually the body's natural defense against an infection in the connective tissues. The body attacks disease agents that cling to the cells or are embedded within them. The infectious agent, and the body's reaction, cause the inflammation, the pain, and the eventual disfigurement of rheumatoid arthritis. When the body makes that response, it also attacks the cell to which the disease agent is connected. But if the agent is taken away, the body immediately stops the attack.

This process differs from true autoimmunity in that one important respect. It can be stopped, and true autoimmunity cannot.

This book is about how those inflammatory forms of arthritis begin, how they operate in the body, and how they can be treated successfully. The last pieces of one of the most complex puzzles in medicine are falling into place.

THE MYTH OF AUTOIMMUNITY

During the long detour, rheumatoid arthritis was treated with drugs that address its symptoms by changing the body's metabolism. The myth of autoimmunity has been used both as the justification for such a drastic approach and as the excuse for its inevitable failure. These drugs are extremely powerful and they will slow down the arthritic reaction, but often at a terrible price; they can damage the retina in the eyes, destroy the marrow in the bones, cause the kidneys to fail, and even kill the patient. One of them, gold, achieved the worst record for mortality of any prescription product on the market.

The reason the effects of metabolic drugs don't endure, so this circular logic goes, is that the autoimmune reaction is unstoppable. The real reason metabolic drugs don't hold up is that they merely mask the symptoms of the disease while they ignore its cause.

Because the prospects seemed so hopeless, doctors have been inclined to ignore the suggestive early symptoms and hope they will go away. Ask anyone you know who suffers from serious rheumatoid arthritis, and the chances are you will hear that it started as a lesser affliction.

Because the autoimmune theory has been taught in most medical schools for the past half-century, rheumatoid arthritis carries with it the stigma of a persistent, downhill condition that can never be cured. Doctors hate that kind of disease, and many of them will diagnose its onset as bursitis, lumbago, tendonitis, polymyositis, synovitis, or osteoarthritis so they can defer dealing with an unstoppable process. That way, a doctor can still do what seems to be best for the patient without having to bring in his heavy artillery such as gold, Plaquenil, chloroquine, penicillamine, Cytoxan, Imuran, or methotrexate to treat the early stages. He can gain a year or two by assuming it's something else.

A THERAPEUTIC PROBE

In their approach to many other diseases, doctors are able to complete a tentative diagnosis by what they call a therapeutic probe. This is the use of a medicine to see if it will relieve a condition—and if it does, the therapy helps verify what the patient is suffering from. But what responsible physician wants to risk inducing blindness or fatal kidney damage just to diagnose or relieve a little bursitis? The doctor has been as badly trapped by the autoimmune theory as his patients.

The infectious view of rheumatoid arthritis has been around far longer than the metabolic theory, but the infectious process is highly complicated, difficult to visualize, and until recently was extremely resistant to the traditional proofs of scientific research. Meanwhile, the metabolic bandwagon achieved such momentum during its forty-year roll, few doctors were aware of alternative treatments.

Today that is no longer the case. In some forms of rheumatoid arthritis the specific infectious agent, such as a mycoplasma or a spirochete, has already been identified. In others it is strongly suspected. There is always a gap in medicine between research results and their application, and most physicians have not yet been trained in dealing with arthritis as an infection—or, more precisely, an infectious allergy or hypersensitivity. But today, instead of prescribing a metabolic drug to suppress the symptoms, if the physician uses the right anti-

CHAPTER 9

Myra Frank

Several years ago I received quite a number of patients from northwest Iowa. The word had gotten around that I had an approach to arthritis that could get results where others didn't, and Myra Frank came to me on such a referral.

Her father called me one morning and asked if I could help his daughter. He said she was twenty-one and desperately ill with rheumatoid arthritis. She had been to the Mayo Clinic where they put her on penicillamine, one of the relatively new drugs at that time; it had the risky component of producing suppression of the bone marrow in some people, and, unfortunately, she was one of the victims of that effect. When he called me, Myra had been sent home, but another hospital had found her white blood cell count was only 700, about 10 percent of what it should be to take care of infection. Ironically, the penicillamine had relieved none of her symptoms before going on to cause this toxic reaction.

I suggested that Mr. Frank take his daughter back to the Mayo Clinic, that they should take responsibility for her condition, but he said Myra refused to go back, that by that time she didn't like doctors at all, she didn't trust them and was thoroughly disillusioned. I made arrangements to get her admitted to the National Hospital at the earliest possible date.

When she arrived, it was obvious that she was every bit as sick as her father had said. She had large, draining abscesses scattered all over her body. Some of them were very deep and went down into the muscle layer. She was obviously frightened and had very little trust of any doctor, including myself. One of my major jobs, I saw at the outset, was to get her to accept some element of hope.

Little by little, we made progress in that direction. She already had been taken off the penicillamine, and the hospital at home had put her on high levels of cortisone in its place; we ended that as well, starting treatment with antibiotics and a low level of steroids to block some of the reaction. She began to pick up. And much to my amazement, her white cells actually began to come up as well.

Generally speaking, when a patient is suffering from aplastic anemia because drugs have stopped the bone marrow from forming cells, the blood levels never come back again and that's the end of it. But Myra's did. I never saw it happen before or since.

Gradually she improved in other ways as well. Eventually, she was healthy enough that one of the plastic surgeons at the hospital began a series of skin transplants to cover the large areas of her backside and leg that had become totally denuded of skin by her reaction to penicillamine.

Then we began to treat her arthritis, which was extremely severe. And that too began to improve.

At each slow step of the way, I could see that we were changing her attitude about medicine and about her disease. We were winning her respect. And most important of all, she was regaining her self-confidence.

Several years have passed. Myra still has active arthritis, but it is easily controlled now under the program. She has had some joint replacements. She has gotten to be strong. She drives a car. She travels around the world. And she has appeared more than once before committees of the Congress of the United States to tell the story of her treatment and recovery. She is an excellent example of someone who has been brought back from a condition that was truly hopeless.

HER STORY

When I was twelve years old, I lived with my parents and two sisters on our farm in Cherokee, Iowa. I was in the seventh grade and very athletic, probably more than even most of the boys in my class. I played every kind of game there was, and I was good at them all. At five feet seven inches and 130 pounds, I was also big for my age, and when we made up teams I was always the first kid my friends and classmates selected to be on their side. One day, a bump appeared on my elbow, and I went to the school nurse. She took one look and told me she thought it was rheumatoid arthritis. That's something old people get, I thought to myself, and I laughed. I had no idea that the childhood I had known was about to end.

The nurse told my parents that I should see our family doctor. When I did, he said the nurse was right about the bump, and he referred me to an arthritis specialist at the University of Iowa Hospital. So we drove six hours to Iowa City, the doctors there told me the same thing I had heard before, and then they sent me home. They didn't seem to be making a big deal out of it, and I didn't think it was a big deal either.

But they kept asking me to come back.

At first, because of my age, I went to pediatrics, but after a year or so they started sending me to rheumatology. By then, if I still had doubts about what lay ahead, all I had to do was look around at the other kids and older patients to get a preview of what was in store. They looked absolutely horrible, and I knew they were really suffering. It was scary, and I'd come out of there feeling very depressed.

My own condition began going downhill fast. My joints ached, and I lost most of my old energy. More subtly, the enthusiasm and hopefulness and excitement for the future that were always a part of my earlier life had drained out of me. I was still at the beginning, still a child, but within those first several months my horizons became shorter and shorter until I deliberately stopped thinking about the future at all. The hospital still hadn't started me on any medication stronger than aspirin, but by the end of the first year I was taking twenty pills a day and that still wasn't enough to do the job. My appetite had fallen off, I had lost twenty pounds, and big knobs started to appear on most of my joints. Because my knee joints began to deteriorate, at a time when my classmates were still growing, I began to get shorter. And I was in pain.

My friends treated me differently, probably because it was so scary for them to see this happening to someone they knew who had been so strong and athletic. In just a few months, I went from being the first one picked to being the last one anyone wanted on his or her team, and that hurt terribly. Pretty soon, I couldn't play at all. I would go to school, come home, and go to bed. I didn't talk to people about my illness. My mother sat down on the edge of my bed one afternoon and asked me to tell her how I felt—not just physically, but how I felt about what was happening to me. I told her I didn't want to talk about it. I wouldn't talk to anyone about it.

There's a lot of height in my family: my father is six feet seven inches, one sister is six feet, and the other sister is five feet ten inches. Both girls are younger than I, but they grew beyond me and eventually became basketball players in high school. I probably would have been tall too, but I stopped growing at the age of thirteen. I suspect the cortisone had something to do with it—my sisters both grew a couple of inches the last two years in high school.

The disease began to affect my marks in school. Through the seventh grade I had been pretty much a straight A student, but when I was a freshman in high school I got my first D. I just didn't have the concentration to study anymore.

During all of these changes, there was one constant: I kept getting in the family car every few months and riding the six hours each way to the hospital in Iowa City. Once I got there, the doctors would seat me on the examining table and shake their heads knowingly about how much worse I was getting, and often a whole team of young doctors or medical students would poke my joints and pull me this way and that. I soon grew to feel that I was making this long journey for the benefit of the doctors, to demonstrate how a disease operates and to reassure them that nature was running its proper course. Once in a while one of them would tell my parents that maybe we would get lucky and the disease would eventually "burn itself out," something that apparently can happen in very rare instances of the juvenile form of the disease. But the condition continued through my adolescence, and it was decided that I didn't have the juvenile form. Never once in the first three years did I hear anyone talk of doing a single thing to make me better.

That changed suddenly during my sophomore year of high school, as I entered the fourth year of the disease. By then I had a lot of joint damage, especially in my hands, and I was badly crippled. On one of my visits to Iowa City, the doctors told me they were going to put me on cortisone. Nobody suggested it would be a cure, but I was told it would help for a while with the symptoms.

The morning after the first treatment I felt so good I almost jumped out of bed. That's the way cortisone is at the beginning. And it wasn't just the first day: it worked well for the next couple of years, and got me back in the mainstream. I look back on cortisone as the reason I was able to get through high school. My grades came back up, and my spirits improved enormously.

I still look back on those high school years as including some very good times. I played drums in the marching band. I attended every athletic event there was, and even though I could no longer participate, I especially loved watching my sisters play basketball. I went to proms and homecoming dances and was in the National Honor Society. And through it all, even though I couldn't bring myself to talk with them about my arthritis, I knew I had a wonderful, loving family behind me.

But cortisone is one of those drugs you're not supposed to take in large quantities or for long periods, and so by the end of my senior year the doctors tried tapering me off. I could never stop cortisone altogether because by this time my body had stopped producing it naturally and I needed to keep up a small maintenance level just to stay alive.

They didn't taper me off in time. I began to develop side effects from the large earlier doses. Most particularly, I began to experience a breakdown of my skin tissue. Every time I banged against something or got a scratch or small puncture, I would develop sores and lesions. My arthritis came back at the same time, even worse than it had been before.

On the strength of my grades during the final three years of high school I enrolled at Iowa State University, but my condition was deteriorating fast. I got a bike so I could cover the sometimes long distances between classes, and I rode it through snow and in all kinds of weather. But I found that the energy I was using to get to class was all the energy I had, and there was nothing left for the work. I would have to sleep on campus a lot, and when I came home to my dorm I was so tired from the return trip that I couldn't study there either. At the end of my second year, I went home to Cherokee for the summer vacation and I got a letter from the school saying I had flunked out. I knew I had worked as hard as I was able, and it was a terrible blow.

Once the doctors had reduced my cortisone, they decided to try injecting me with gold. I can't remember now what the treatments cost, but they were terribly expensive. One of the side effects of gold can be kidney failure, and a first indicator that the gold is attacking the kidneys is protein in the urine. The protein showed up in tests after just a few months, and so the gold was stopped. It hadn't seemed to do a thing to improve my arthritis, and when they stopped giving it to me I didn't feel any different either.

The doctors switched to Plaquenil, which had been developed initially to fight malaria. Although I developed no side effects, I also showed no signs that it was doing my arthritis any good, so after six months they stopped that treatment as well and switched back to gold. All together, I was on the gold for about a year, until they had to stop it permanently. By this time I was feeling very sick. I had no energy, was seriously anemic, in a lot of pain, and very depressed. I also had the feeling that I should be trying harder, but I just didn't have the energy to do more than I did. And I didn't like my family and friends to have to see what I was going through, so I made an effort to pretend that everything was fine. That strategy didn't fool anyone around me—it was perfectly obvious that I was in terrible shape—but because I spent so much time pretending, I never was able to come to terms with what was really happening to me.

I did have some good friends who stuck by me, and I often wondered what they were thinking—about me, about my disease, and about how I was handling myself. In a way, thinking about their reactions was as close as I dared get to thinking about where my life was going.

When I had left college I was majoring in accounting, so I enrolled in a small technical school in Sheldon, about fifty miles from home, and tried to resume my studies. But it didn't work. It seemed as though trying to lead a normal, productive life only made the arthritis worse, and the more I ignored it, the more it demanded my attention. The problem wasn't just the arthritis; the side effects were getting more serious at the same time.

I began to lose skin. A large sore appeared on my rear, and new sores emerged on my fingers, all exuding pus and causing a lot of discomfort. My white blood cell count dropped steeply, so my body's ability to heal itself and its natural defense against infections were very weak. All these problems were explained as the natural side effects of cortisone and the other drugs I'd been given, and the doctors kept saying they wanted me to get off the cortisone—but they didn't know how to do it.

We decided it was time to try something different, so I left the university hospital in Iowa City and started seeing a doctor in Omaha, Nebraska. My dad was usually the one to make those decisions; I really didn't care one way or another. I didn't have a whole lot of hope that anyone was ever going to find any way to help me, and I guess I was getting pretty dejected about going back to places where we spent a lot of money and no one could tell us anything.

Even so, I still wasn't totally cynical about the doctors who had been treating me. During the whole course of the disease, a lot of people would approach me or my family and ask if we had tried carrot juice or cod liver oil or whatever the latest fad was, and we'd see stories in the newspapers at the supermarket checkouts about exotic cures of one kind or another, but we just ignored them all. I continued to believe that the doctors who had studied the disease would know about every treatment on the market, and that if they didn't tell me about it, it was because it didn't work.

I had an appointment to see the doctor in Omaha one Monday morning, so I came home from school in Sheldon the Friday before in order to spend the weekend with my family in Cherokee. It had been normal for me to run a fever of 100 or 101 over the previous year, and my weight had dropped to just around a hundred pounds. My dress was a size 5. I felt sick most of the time. That Sunday night, as we were all sitting at the dining room table after dinner, for no apparent reason and without any warning, I suddenly vomited. It happened again a short time later in the kitchen.

In addition to being slightly embarrassed, I felt even worse than usual. We knew I was going to see the doctor the next day, so after a while I sat in an easy chair beside the telephone, trying to get my mind off the way I felt by studying. My father recalls that a short time later he was reading in the living room, and when he heard me talking in the dining room, he assumed I was using the phone. Then he realized that I was mumbling incoherently, and when he came out to the dining room he found me bent over the side of the chair in convulsions. I don't remember anything until I woke up in the emergency room of our local hospital. They stopped the convulsions and put me in an ambulance to Omaha.

The doctors in Omaha stayed up with me all night, running tests, trying to find out what had happened. What they finally determined was that an infection from all the sores on my body had suddenly "turned on," and that my temperature had shot up to 105 as my system tried to fight it, producing the convulsions.

They gave me antibiotics to fight the infection. They also decided I needed to put on weight and they put me on a 4,000-calorie diet. I didn't gain any weight to speak of, and although the infection seemed to eventually diminish, the doctors were unable to heal the lesions. After a month in the hospital they sent me home, still covered with sores.

I went back to the technical college, but I knew by then that my further education was a lost cause and that I was going to have to stay close to home, because I couldn't take care of myself. Shortly afterward I saw an ad for a bookkeeper in Cherokee, and I resigned from the school and moved back in with my family.

During the following year, the side effects were always with me, and even though I managed to work fairly steadily on the new job, I had the feeling that I was sitting on a deadly bomb and that it was just about to explode. I had sores on the bottoms of my feet, and at the end of that year one of my feet suddenly began to swell. I knew that once more, the bomb was going off.

It was the weekend of a family reunion, and I just wasn't up to attending, so I stayed at home in bed. Dad must have been doing a lot of thinking about it, because when everyone came back, he walked into my bedroom and said, "What do you think about going up to Rochester, Minnesota, to the Mayo Clinic?"

I could feel the tears coming into my eyes. I was so sick of those places I never wanted to see another one. Each new hospital was a little farther away than the last, and I knew that none of them could do anything for me. I told him I was sure the Mayo Clinic would be just one more place where I was a guinea pig for the doctors to poke and probe, and that I'd get nothing out of it.

But as usual I said yes.

The doctors up at Mayo examined me thoroughly, and then told me it was time to try something a little different. They had a new drug called penicillamine.

I recognized the name. It was all the rage at the time; I had seen an article about it in the *National Enquirer* and knew that penicillamine had gone through the FDA double-blind study and showed great promise. But I also knew that cortisone and gold and Plaquenil and untold numbers of other "wonder drugs" had similarly gone through the double-blind tests with flying colors in their times, only to eventually fail badly in sustained clinical use. I agreed without much enthusiasm or hope, and the Mayo Clinic began yet another course of treatment.

While I was in Rochester, right at the beginning of the penicillamine therapy, a new sore erupted on my leg. It was only about the size of a quarter at the beginning, but it was really deep and was extremely painful. Meanwhile, the doctors at Mayo examined the sore on my rear that had been open for the past two years and decided to do a skin graft. The skin was so unhealthy that the graft failed. And the sore on my leg got deeper and more painful.

My white blood count was very low when I arrived in Rochester, and I was kept in isolation for the entire duration of my stay. Rochester was a long way for anyone to travel from Cherokee—about seven hours by car—and so my family only got up there a few times during the first month, and I had one or two visits from a girlfriend I'd known since high school who had stuck with me through everything. One day the doctor came in and told me that I could expect to be in there for another three or four months. When he left I cried and cried, and no matter how much I wanted to stop I couldn't turn off the tears.

I had plenty of time to think while I lay there in isolation; I wasn't allowed to get out of bed even to go to the bathroom. I didn't like the way my life was going. I couldn't even bring myself to consider the future, but I knew in the back of my mind that the day was going to come soon when I would be truly helpless, and I would be dependent on someone else to take care of me. If I had any doubts, they were dispelled one day when a hospital social worker or psychologist came into my room and started to counsel me on how to accept my disease. She told me I could expect to be in a wheelchair in the not-too-distant future. I think she was feeling me out to determine how realistic I was about what lay ahead.

My father was visiting with me at the time she appeared, and I noticed during her little talk that he turned white as a sheet. Perhaps her remarks had been for his benefit as well, because certainly what she was telling me would have an impact on the whole family. As for me, instead of being shocking, the revelation was a matter of real indifference; I didn't think of myself as being a part of life at that point anyway, and I listened to her with no particular reaction. When she left the room, I realized with some surprise that my father was furious. "Don't listen to a word she said," he told me. "She doesn't know what she's talking about."

Soon after that, my father decided on another, completely different course of action. He came up one weekend in the middle of my second month and told me about a story he had seen in an Iowa newspaper, during the same family reunion when he had heard about the Mayo Clinic. The article was about a rheumatoid arthritic named Don Knop, a young college student from Iowa who had gone to the National Hospital outside Washington and been treated by a doctor named Thomas McPherson Brown. It said Knop's arthritis was now under control, that he was able to function normally with no exotic chemicals and no side effects. When my father showed me the clipping, I read it quickly and let it drop on the bed, then turned my face away and stared out the window at the construction going on outside in a world I didn't seem to be a part of. I was certain this was just one more beginning of another painful and inevitable defeat. It was more than I could bear.

My father patiently explained that he had learned far more about the story than was in the newspaper. He said he had met the Knop family and had heard of their son's experience at first hand. He had even listened to a tape recording that Dr. Brown had given them on the nature of their son's disease, its prognosis under the treatment he had begun, and the course it would follow to its conclusion.

"Conclusion" was a word I had never heard before in the whole decade of my ordeal. It didn't inspire the least bit of hope, but I realized when my father said it that no one ever before had talked about the possibility of my disease coming to an end. Dad went on and on; he was filled with excitement, and he was trying to pass some of it to me.

But instead of the reaction he was looking for, all he got from me was tears. He asked if I could explain why I was crying, and all I could say, over and over, was, "I don't know. I don't know."

But looking back on it, I think I do. I usually cried only when I was facing a new treatment or hospital. Maybe it forced me to think of the future. After ten years of torture and heartbreak, I had become terrified of hope; I knew where it would lead. I couldn't bear to consider the possibility that he might be right.

Two things happened during that visit. My father finally got me to agree to go to Washington to meet Dr. Brown, with whom he had already made an appointment. And, because the doctors apparently couldn't think of anything else to do with me, I was told to "go home and wait it out"; so I left the Mayo Clinic.

Because I was still continuing the penicillamine therapy, arrangements were made for me to have my blood and urine tested every two weeks at our local hospital for toxicity.

The trip to Washington was scheduled for about ninety days after my release from Mayo, on the twelfth of December. About a month before that date, I went into our hospital for the regular biweekly tests, and when I returned home I felt really sick. There was nothing alarming in this, because I felt sick almost all the time. I went to my room and lay down on the bed. I hadn't been lying there for more than a few minutes when the phone rang; it was the doctor who monitored the tests, telling my mother she had to get me back to the hospital as soon as possible. My white count had dropped to 700, which is very, very bad. In fact, they were afraid they might not be able to get it back up again.

My parents remember the times they visited me during the next couple of days while I was in isolation; my skin was gray, and they were frightened that I wasn't going to make it. The simple act of turning slightly in the bed produced pure agony. For the first time, I sensed the possibility that I might be about to die.

The local doctor ended the penicillamine therapy immediately, then raised my cortisone to an extremely high level; a little later my white count began to rise in response. The crisis passed. I stayed off the penicillamine, which should never have been prescribed for me in the first place with my low white count, and a month later I went to Washington.

I met Dr. Brown. We talked for a long time, and he explained to me how arthritis occurs; it was the first time anyone had discussed my illness with me in terms of its cause. He then explained what he was going to do to help me, and why simple antibiotic therapy would work. That was another first; no one else had discussed results, because in no previous treatment had positive results been a realistic possibility. At the end of that first meeting I was finally able to look at the future for the first time in ten years, not as something to be feared, but with hope.

I stayed at the hospital for less than a month, and by the time I went home I could already feel the difference. I had more energy. I was no longer smothered by depression. I felt better. My lesions and sores closed and began at last to heal. I had some skin grafts, and this time they worked. A few months later, I felt well enough to return to school—not at the technical college near my home, but back at Iowa State.

I graduated in 1983 with a degree in accounting. That September I got a job as an auditor with the Army Audit Agency, an opening I heard about from someone I met at the National Hospital, and I just recently moved to a similar job with the Office of the Inspector General. In just those few months, the world opened up to me again and I walked back into it.

I wrote to most of the doctors who had treated me since I was a child and told them about the astonishing thing that had finally happened. I gave them all the information about the causes and mechanism of arthritis that I had learned from Dr. Brown and from scientific papers that he and other researchers have published in medical journals. I described the treatment and my recovery. I felt my greatest responsibility now was to pass along the secret of new life for use on other patients they might treat for the same disease.

Several doctors wrote back. A rheumatologist from the Mayo Clinic told me that this kind of thing happens now and then in rheumatoid arthritis, and that nobody really knows why—it's just a matter of timing. He suggested that my treatment in Washington probably had nothing to do with my getting well. A doctor in Iowa City told me there was no scientific proof for the treatment I had received at the Arthritis Institute, and he said that such proof could only be derived from six-month double-blind studies—the same studies through which the drugs that nearly killed me had all passed with flying colors before displaying any of their lethal effects. Both letters made me very angry.

The doctor from Omaha was an internist, not a rheumatologist, and he wrote back too. He said he had heard of Dr. Brown and was very interested in how things were going; he asked me to keep him posted. Unlike the other two doctors, he wasn't defending an entrenched position, and he was willing to listen to his patient. I felt he really cared.

I remember a few of the other things I heard about rheumatoid arthritis from the Mayo Clinic and from a lot of other doctors and hospitals, and I have the choice of believing those things or believing my own experience. And I'm not alone; I met and talked with many other patients whose arthritis has been brought under control or into complete remission by Dr. Brown's treatment—there are over ten thousand of them. Today I don't sit in a wheelchair, and I don't expect I ever will. Instead, I have a wonderful, productive career and travel all over the world.

I have a life.

At last.

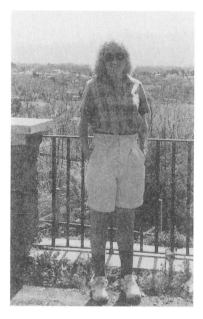

Myra Frank, who lost her childhood to juvenile RA, now travels the world as a government auditor for the Inspector General's Office (the picture was taken just outside Rome.) The story of Myra's treatment and recovery was the first case history in *The Road Back* (chapter 9 of this book); a decade later, her name became a fitting homophone for the NIH-sponsored MIRA trials, which vindicated the therapy that saved her life.

Talmadge Williams, Ph.D., educator and consultant in Arlington, Va., was another of Dr. Brown's patients. His case history appears in chapter 13 of this book. When Dr. Williams was interviewed about his recovery on the television program "20/20," on camera he picked up a packing case containing a heavy computer printer and, with little apparent effort, placed it on his office shelf.

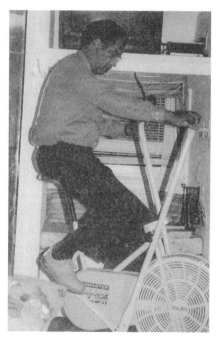

The Golden Calf and Other Stories

Most physicians who treat arthritis tell their patients that there is a certain amount of risk in whatever medication they prescribe, but that there is a bigger risk in the disease. There are two important things, however, that most doctors *don't* tell their patients about that same medication.

They don't tell them that it will end up curing the disease or stopping its progress. Because it won't.

They don't tell them that the medication will eventually wear out, that it will stop working. But it will.

If the patient is incurring a serious risk by taking a drug that will wear out, that is a very different thing from taking the same risk with a medicine that will keep on working or that offers an outside chance of sustaining control. None of the traditional drugs prescribed for rheumatoid arthritis has an outside chance of sustaining control, and not one has ever cured a single case. All drugs that have been created specifically for treating arthritis eventually lose their effectiveness. That's why there are so many of them: the drug companies have to keep on bringing out something new to replace the previous drugs as they give out.

In the late 1970s, at the World Congress of Rheumatology in San Francisco, I gave a paper suggesting the joint scan as a means of determining whether the various forms of medication were helping to improve patient health; it was the first proposal for an objective measure of drug efficacy. Coincidentally, at the very same time that paper was presented, penicillamine was announced as the new drug that would cure arthritis. Penicillamine had been a big hit in England, and it got a lot of attention in the American press as a result. And no one paid the slightest attention to the proposal that we establish a scientific means for determining whether these drugs were really doing all the things that were being claimed for them.

Of course, the other thing our paper showed was that tetracycline did indeed produce improvements that were measurable in the joint scans, and that those improvements endured.

Two years later, the discovery was made that penicillamine produced aplastic anemia, and its luster began to diminish. In fact, by the time penicillamine was introduced in the United States, the medical community in England was already becoming aware that there could be some slight problems with it—that its benefits didn't last, and that its other effects were potentially lethal. But while they were waking up to these horrors on one side of the Atlantic, the medical world was celebrating this same product as the new Silver Bullet on the other.

SLIPPING BY THE DOUBLE-BLIND

Most of the troubles with these wonder cures appear late, usually just past the six-month double-blind testing period. As a result, the screening agencies that are supposed to be watching these things have left the job, and nobody monitors the changes that are taking place. The literature is already out, and it gives the impression of a sustained improvement because the drug worked for the first six months and everyone assumes that the trend will continue on the same upward curve. In reality, what happens instead is that the curve almost inevitably goes down. With tetracycline, on the other hand, I have not seen any toxic effects in forty years in anybody. The drug is used in low doses, widely spaced to avoid sensitization; the higher the physician has to go in dosage, the wider the spaces. Extreme cases can be treated intravenously, which avoids potential allergic responses by going into a part of the body where allergies don't take place. Tetracycline doesn't attack the part of germs where immunity is formed, so it can be used virtually forever without giving rise to immune strains of the organism it is fighting.

Because of these features, I have been able to treat patients from Washington or Texas or California or Alaska or Cairo, get them started on tetracycline therapy, and then send them back home to continue a program of no-risk recovery. All they need is some help from their family doctor, and it has been my experience that in most cases such doctors are very glad to learn of the technique and see it through to a successful conclusion. If there are any problems with a tetracycline patient going out of balance and his dosage needing to be changed, the doctor can call me back or make the adjustment on his own, but there is never any risk whatever of a toxic effect. Indeed, a lot of physicians continue to use the same technique on other sufferers from rheumatoid arthritis, so the benefits spread.

By comparison, it would be extremely questionable practice for a physician who was treating someone with gold or methotrexate, for example, to let the patient out of his sight for any longer than a few days, such as for a trip abroad or even a short vacation in another state. Things happen too quickly with that kind of medication. With gold, the main risks are damage to the kidneys and bone marrow and destruction of the process by which the body creates platelets. In Germany, the use of oral gold in the treatment of arthritis has been identified as the cause of platelet depression in two cases where the patient subsequently bled to death from a simple bruise.

Methotrexate is an anticancer drug that was designed to interfere with the immune system. Like cortisone, it produces its effect by blocking the antigen-antibody reaction, but also like cortisone it leaves the antigen ready to react again. It is an extremely toxic compound which can damage the liver and the lungs, and sooner or later the physician has to stop giving it. Meanwhile, the patient has started on a journey similar to the one on which Moses led the Israelites through the Red Sea. The waters part for a time, but the path is inevitably downward and the risk of drowning from the walls of water on either side increases with each successive step. No physician who has entered this course has ever proven to be as wise or as successful as Moses; no one has gotten a single patient across to the Promised Land.

RISKS VS. BENEFITS

This type of medicine gains its advantage through a much larger disadvantage, and its risks are immense. The advantage is short-term pain relief. The disadvantages are severe whiplash as the arthritis mechanism gathers new fury once the treatment is stopped, along with the strong possibility of destruction of the lungs, and of liver damage that can lead to uremia and death. (A 1987 study of the efficacy and safety of methotrexate therapy in rheumatoid arthritis at McMaster University in Ontario by Tugwell, Bennett, and Gent cites nausea, vomiting, anorexia, and diarrhea in 10 percent of the subjects surveyed, stomatitis in 6 percent, leukopenia, anemia, or thrombocytopenia in 3 percent, and "rare" instances of toxicity of the liver, kidneys, or lungs, possible malignancy, oligospermia, fever, gynecomastia, localized osteoporosis, and leukocytonbastic vasculitis. Therapy had to be discontinued in one-third of those surveyed because of these and other effects. Their conclusion? "If approved [by the FDA], the drug should be given to patients with rheumatoid arthritis refractory to first- and second-line agents, such as injectable gold and penicillamine, who provide informed consent.")

HANDICAPPING THE DOCTOR

The liabilities of these products place an enormous burden on the rheumatologists who use them, a burden which shifts the attention of the physician away from the disease and focuses it instead on monitoring the high-risk treatment. With those drugs that impair platelet formation, that monitoring can take the form of periodic checks of the bone marrow, a process which is not only very costly but extremely painful. And of course it keeps the patient on a very short tether.

A method of treatment which does not entail those liabilities of great risk, pain, expense, and inconvenience, on the other hand, frees both the doctor and the patient from the need for close monitoring. A general physician doesn't have the time to follow his patient as closely as a rheumatologist, but with tetracycline he doesn't have to. When I order a blood test for a patient on a program of antibiotic therapy, it isn't to see whether the patient is surviving the medication, but rather to measure factors such as sedimentation rate or hemoglobin level to determine our progress in combating the disease of arthritis.

Once more, the only treatment that has any hope of curing rheumatoid arthritis is one that addresses the cause. Treatments that deal with the problem by placing the symptoms in a state of suspension are doomed to fail over the long term, and often at a terrible price. Antibiotic therapy is the only approach that dries up the source. It may require great persistence on the part of both the doctor and the patient, but I don't believe there is any possible shortcut, now or in the future.

The number of arthritics in the population mounts each

year. Just a couple of years ago it was 34 million, and now it has risen to 37 million. About half those people suffer from straight rheumatoid arthritis, and if you add in the patients who are afflicted with a combination of rheumatoid and osteoarthritis, the number is at least 25 million.

OSTEOARTHRITIS IS DIFFERENT

Osteoarthritis is a noninflammatory form of arthritis that is hereditary and is considered to be incurable. It is characterized by calcium deposits which can accumulate on pressure points and impinge on nerves, so there is some pain associated with it, although it is different from the pain that goes with the rheumatoid form. I have found that as a rule, when an osteoarthritis patient complains bitterly about the disease, it is because there is a component of rheumatoid arthritis mixed in with it. Until fairly recently it was very difficult to demonstrate the presence of rheumatoid arthritis in that kind of combination, because the osteo obscured the picture. However, the bone and joint scan has greatly illuminated the picture in recent times by revealing inflammatory reactions associated with the calcium pressure points.

This population of perhaps 10 million arthritics who have both forms represents a major added challenge, because a safe method of treatment is needed to allow the physician to probe therapeutically. It makes no sense to probe a possible combination of osteo and rheumatoid with gold or penicillamine or Plaquenil because the drugs are so dangerous to begin with. Until the bone scanner came along, many physicians chose to deal with the problem by concluding it wasn't there: they said that there was no such combination, and that a patient had either osteo or rheumatoid but never both. We have found through our own use of the bone scanner and tests for the mycoplasma antibody that approximately half the cases of osteoarthritis involve some degree of the rheumatoid form.

TOWARD PREVENTION

One of the great advantages of the tetracycline approach is that it allows the use of a safe therapeutic probe early in the disease when the risks from many of the standard drugs outweigh their possible usefulness. Early treatment is far more effective than late management. The antibiotic approach has already opened the way for treatment to prevent arthritis.

CHAPTER 11

Lauriane Riley

(As told by her mother)

About a year ago, when Lauriane was two years old, she developed a fever and a rash. The fever came and went intermittently for about fourteen days, and she was tired a lot and lost her appetite, so we finally put her into the local hospital. Some tests were done, and the doctor told us she was suffering from juvenile rheumatoid arthritis.

Our first question was how serious was it, and the doctors said they didn't know, that we'd have to wait and see. It was a frustrating time. They prepared us for the worst, telling us that this was a crippling disease, but they couldn't really tell us anything tangible about *how* crippling, or how soon it would happen, and they sent her home after four days.

Lauriane had a little stiffness in her knees, and the doctors told us to watch them for swelling and unusual warmth. They prescribed aspirin, but the dosage soon proved too much for her stomach so we had to cut way back.

In the meantime, I spoke with a friend, Dr. Cecil Jacobson, and he told me about Dr. Brown at the Arthritis Institute. He encouraged me to get a second opinion, and if it agreed with the first to take Lauriane to the Arthritis Institute.

For the second opinion we went to a large hospital in Washington. They confirmed the original diagnosis and were even more pessimistic about what we could expect for Lauriane's future. While we were at the second hospital, I mentioned to the doctors there that we were considering taking her to Dr. Brown. They said they had heard of him, but they didn't say anything else, good or bad. I have a lot of respect for Dr. Jacobson, who is a well-known geneticist, and even though he does not specialize in arthritis I trusted his referral, so I didn't press the Washington doctors to say anything more.

Lauriane and I met with Dr. Brown two days later at the National Hospital. By that time her legs had started to become stiff, she was reluctant to walk, her sedimentation rate was abnormally high, and she was suffering from anemia. Dr. Brown treated her with small doses of oral antibiotic and within three weeks all of those symptoms had disappeared. Six months later, in a complete laboratory workup at the National Hospital, not a single sign of arthritis remained.

A year has passed since Dr. Brown treated Lauriane. She has not had a fever since he started the medication, and there is no trace of stiffness in her legs or any reluctance to do all of the normal things—running, playing—that healthy children do. She eats well, has grown normally, and has lots of energy. She is completely recovered.

CHAPTER 12.

The Case for Early Detection and Treatment

W hen an earthquake is about to take place, something happens in nature that prefigures the coming cataclysm. Dogs howl, cats climb trees, and birds stop singing. Whatever it is that signals these other members of the animal kingdom, man alone remains oblivious to the warning, either because he can't detect it, or because he doesn't recognize its meaning. Nature provides similar advance notice of the advent of diseases. Over the years, it has become clear that there is a forerunner to the development of acute rheumatoid arthritis, and in taking histories and treating patients, I have learned to become suspicious when certain symptoms are mentioned.

FATIGUE: THE EARLY WARNING

The most important of all antecedents to the rheumatoid explosion, the first development symptom on which one can most reliably base the suspicion that rheumatoid arthritis is about to happen, is unexplained fatigue; it precedes almost every case I have ever treated, sometimes coming on a year before there is any particular discomfort in the joints.

The fatigue will be serious enough that the patient goes to the doctor, but the doctor doesn't know what he is looking for and as a rule he doesn't find anything. He tells the patient that he or she is working too hard or is under too much stress. Another gambit is to ask the patient's age, and then to suggest that when one gets to that point in life—whatever point it happens to be—one naturally slows down a bit. That way, the doctor can sound profound at the same time as he admits his ignorance, which is precisely the posture favored by most physicians when they haven't the foggiest idea what's happening.

The patient starts to become anxious; feeling tired and poorly is bad enough, but not knowing why is worse. Perhaps there is something else going on. Or perhaps, as the doctor seems to suggest, the patient expects too much from life or is not altogether balanced psychologically. People who are tired are also down emotionally, so these suggestions fall on fertile soil.

ANEMIA AND OTHER SIGNS

Sometimes the fatigue is accompanied by anemia, and the physician usually jumps at the chance to connect the two as effect and cause. And when he finds that the anemia doesn't respond to iron or vitamin B-12 or folic acid or liver or to any of the things that ordinarily tend to raise the blood count, the common stratagem is to blame the intransigence of the anemia on the patient's peculiar nature, which, in turn, adds to the patient's anxiety. Stress has been clearly identified as an accelerator of the disease process, so by now the doctor has become a part of the problem.

When the next symptom emerges, it is usually a troublesome joint. The common reaction at this point is for the doctor to diagnose it as a sprain, and when the patient can't recall any event that might explain such a result, the doctor blames it on the patient's faulty memory. The diagnosis seems to be vindicated when the joint pain subsides and disappears, as usually happens with these first small warning shots before the arthritis explodes.

We have found that when a patient first complains of fatigue, especially if there is any connection with joint complaints, a test of blood for mycoplasma antibodies will produce positive results. Moreover, many patients will display these results for mycoplasma antibodies when nothing else shows. I have reached the conclusion, through long experience in following thousands of such patients, that even in the absence of any other indicator, signs of mycoplasmas in the blood are a guarantee that the patient is eventually going to develop either rheumatoid arthritis or some other disease of the connective tissue unless treatment is started. And I have learned not to wait.

THE IMPORTANCE OF HISTORY

At this stage it is also possible to gain supporting evidence by going back into the patient's history. Many have had periods of fatigue before, and some can recall times when they were also suffering from depression, although most people have never spoken of the depression to anyone or looked at it from the viewpoint that it might be a symptom of something else. There is a certain amount of risk in admitting to either fatigue or depression, and most people would rather accept these symptoms as normal parts of growing up than take that risk in bringing them out for examination. I suspect that in most such cases, the fatigue and depression go back to early childhood.

Of course there are other disorders that can explain fatigue—such as mononucleosis, infectious hepatitis, or low thyroid function—and these should be on the physician's list of things to eliminate. But once they have been ruled out, the doctor should be suspicious of early rheumatoid disease, and not write it off as an emotional imbalance. This is particularly important because at the time the fatigue develops, the patient is also usually more tense and nervous. These traits may owe to natural worry about a symptom that cannot be explained, or they may be symptoms in themselves, as we know them to be at later stages of rheumatoid disease.

Many other psychological factors can appear in this early syndrome of arthritis: irritability, reduced mental acuity, slower motor skills, shorter attention span, hesitancy, and loss of confidence. These can be bothersome to anybody, but they are particularly frightening to older people, who often interpret them as early signs of senility or Alzheimer's disease.

Some pre-arthritics are extraordinarily sensitive to cold. I had one patient arrive in my office wearing a fur coat on a hot summer day. Others can be overly sensitive to heat. An impaired thermostat in either direction is a warning sign.

THE ATTACK

When the actual rheumatoid aspect finally shows itself, it is most commonly first seen in the small joints of the hands, feet, and ankles, although not always by any means. Regardless of where it begins, the real key to early rheumatoid disease is its migratory nature; it is an elusive Gypsy. Many people are misled by that nomadic feature into the belief that once it has left a particular area, it has cleared up. But it always comes back, becoming progressively more constant and more fixed.

From a treatment point of view, once the disease starts becoming localized, it is getting more serious. The migratory phase, before the body has started to encase the infectious agent inside its defensive walls of scars and inflammation, is considerably simpler to get at.

That is pretty much the way rheumatoid arthritis starts. In some cases it can tarry at one or another of these stages for months or even a few years, slight, insidious, mistaken for something else, often simply tolerated and ignored. In other cases it can explode overnight with a violence that leaves its victim suffering agonies in every joint.

It is interesting that people who experience an explosive onset often go into remission for a couple of years. Their immune systems have been shaken up to fight back hard, and protect them for a period following the attack. This action and reaction portrays a typical infectious process, and even when the arthritis finally returns after that kind of a start, it is frequently more responsive to treatment than the kind that seems to creep into the system a little bit at a time.

Viral pneumonia is a good prototype for what happens when a mycoplasma infection becomes fixed around a certain area. In the lung, the disease produces sections of what look like nodules of granulation material, inflamed tissues that are apparently fixed around the infectious organism and remain in position for months, producing the characteristic cough of the disease. I visualize the same thing happening in the joints, although it's a lot harder to see there; we seldom biopsy joint tissue, although doctors used to, because we have found that rheumatoid arthritis tends to produce excessive scars where the mycoplasmas cluster, and the biopsy produces more pain than the information is worth.

LETTING THE BODY DEFEND ITSELF

The physician has to pay careful attention to the body's defense mechanism as one of the primary aspects of the treatment of rheumatoid arthritis. He has to let the body do as much as it can to suppress the agents that cause the arthritis. That means carefully reducing the barriers which the body erects around the mycoplasmas so that they can be effectively purged without stimulating the production of the toxins that characterize the allergic flareup.

The doctor starts this process on first seeing the patient by giving some simple anti-inflammatory remedy such as aspirin, Bufferin, Ecotrin, or the like, the choice depending on how the patient's stomach responds; this assumes the disease is a fresh, new case and not severe. (I must admit that only about 5 percent of the patients in my own practice are in this category; as a rule, by the time a patient gets as far as the Arthritis Institute, the disease is pretty well advanced.) The purpose in using these mild anti-inflammatories is not to treat symptoms, but rather to permit the body to get through its own barriers. If the aspirin doesn't do the job, the doctor goes on to the encids: Clinoril, Naprosyn, Meclomen, Tolectin, Nalfon, Motrin, or similar drugs.

The doctor has to be continuously mindful of the mechanism, and not the symptoms, when he is treating the disease. This calls for a clear understanding of a very complex process (described in detail in Chapter 18) and a certain degree of tough-mindedness. The physician's main responsibility is to relieve the disease, not just to make the patient feel better without regard for what happens next.

CHAPTER 13

Talmadge Williams, Ph.D.

My problem started back in the middle seventies. I was working for a computer firm, and when I went for my annual physical checkup the doctor told me that the blood test had revealed traces of rheumatoid arthritis. I hadn't noticed any symptoms that would have made me suspect there was anything seriously wrong; in fact, the only unusual thing I could recall was minor—a slight tingling or numbness occasionally at the ends of my fingers—but no pain and no stiffness. The doctor took the blood test seriously, however, and sent me over to George Washington University Hospital.

The tests were repeated at the hospital, the new doctor confirmed the signs of arthritis, and I was given some pills and sent home. The pills were Naprosyn, an anti-inflammatory analgesic, which I was to take just a couple of times a week. I followed the hospital's directions for the next couple of years, and everything seemed to be fine.

One night I was sitting at my desk at home, studying for my work; I had to concentrate hard on learning about changes in my field of employment, which seemed to occur almost daily. Moreover, I was under a lot of family stress at the time. As I idly scratched my head during the study session that particular evening, I felt something sticky and, when I withdrew my hand, discovered blood on my fingers. In looking at the mirror a moment later, I saw that I had scratched a small hole in my scalp. I was annoyed with myself, but not at all alarmed. I interpreted the event as an indicator of the stress I was under, and nothing more.

After a few days, the hair around the lesion still had not started to grow back and I became concerned. I made an appointment with a dermatologist at Howard University Hospital and was given some salve, Lindex ointment, to help restore the hair. The doctor didn't exaggerate the problem of a small, self-inflicted scratch on my head, but he was more concerned with why it had happened so easily and why the hair had not come back on its own. He asked me about my medical history, and I told him about the rheumatoid arthritis. As soon as he heard that, he sent me over to see their rheumatologist.

The rheumatologist did some more tests, and the next day he called me and said, "Williams, you have lupus." He had me come back in, prescribed some medication, and the next day I was extremely sick. I decided it was time for me to head back to George Washington Hospital to talk with the doctor who had diagnosed my arthritis two years earlier.

Back at GW, my original doctor ran the standard tests again and told me I did not have lupus, but that my skin problem was related to the arthritis and it was time to change my treatment. He increased the amount of Naprosyn to twice the dosage, now taken three times every day. The condition quickly began to get worse. I saw swelling in my ankles and wrists, nodules came up on my elbow and wrist, and I started to become very stiff. He saw that the original medicine wasn't doing the job, so he decided to put me on gold.

The gold treatment consisted of fifty milligrams injected in my muscles every week. Each time I went over for the shot, they gave me blood and urine tests beforehand to make sure I wasn't having a reaction. The treatment was very costly— something in the neighborhood of $140 every week, plus the time away from my job. The plan was that I would take the shots weekly for about three months, then it would be every other week for a while, and then eventually every month. But after about the tenth week I had deteriorated so badly that when I went in for my weekly shot they gave me a cane.

Things continued to go downhill. Over the next few years, my ankles became so badly swollen the doctor began talking to me about a wheelchair. I had nodules on both elbows, and was in a lot of pain. I stayed on the gold but moved from one anti-inflammatory medication to another, staying with each one until I developed the inevitable reaction, then moving on to something else in the same family.

Friends told me about different things they had heard of that were supposed to help arthritis, and in particular I began to be careful about what I ate. I eliminated chocolate, processed meats that contained a lot of animal fats and gristle like hot dogs and bologna, sugar—I kept hearing about new things to avoid, and I'd cut them out of my life. None of this seemed to have any impact whatsoever, and I kept looking for something new, something that might help me.

And that's how I happened to be looking through the paper one day when I saw a story about a gorilla. The gorilla had serious arthritis, and a doctor at the National Hospital had cured him. I thought to myself, "If this Dr. Brown can do that for a gorilla, I should think he could do something for me." So I picked up the telephone.

The lady who answered at the Arthritis Clinic told me there was a waiting list of somewhere around six months. I thanked her, and hung up. I'm a salesman, and I know how to get past the receptionist in just about any organization I've ever seen, so I called again at a few minutes past five, and Dr. Brown himself answered the telephone. When I finished talking with him, he told me to come in the next day.

I think the thing that decided him was hearing that I was on gold. He told me he was very much opposed to gold, and that he could help me with the arthritis. He outlined in very exact detail what he planned to do for me, and then afterward he gave me a written copy of everything he had said. I told him I wanted to think it over, but that I'd let him know in a few days.

My next stop was George Washington Hospital, where I showed Dr. Brown's paper to the rheumatologist who had been treating me from the onset of the disease. He looked at Dr. Brown's plan for a moment or two, and a little smile came to his face. He told me he knew Dr. Brown, and that he liked him a lot and respected him. He also said he knew of Dr. Brown's theory. He made it clear to me that he did not personally oppose the theory, but he said the problem was that it had not been proven. Finally, he said, "Something tells me you're going to try Dr. Brown's treatment anyway, Mr. Williams, regardless of whatever I might tell you."

I tried to analyze what it all meant. There was nothing mean or disparaging in anything the doctor said; in fact, the tone was positive and friendly, and I felt a little bit as though I had discovered a secret which the doctor already knew but still couldn't acknowledge. I decided that was my answer, so I said, "I'm going to give Dr. Brown's treatment a trial of six months. But if it gets me into trouble and I have a lot of pain, I want you to promise that you'll take me back as a patient. And by the same token, if it seems that after six months I'm getting better, I want you to do a full series of tests and take X rays so you can tell me if the improvement is real or imaginary."

The doctor agreed, and we parted on good terms.

I went over to the Arthritis Clinic and started Dr. Brown's treatment. There were no injections; everything was oral. I expected the results to take a long time to show, but within no more than three weeks the improvement was astonishing. The swelling started to go down, I was able to move around without hobbling, I got rid of the cane, and I felt better than I had felt in years.

What also happened was that my medical expenses dropped from $140 a week, which is what I had been paying for the dangerous drugs that didn't work, to about $35 a month for safe medicine that did. I've had a long time to think about why the medical establishment refuses to accept Dr. Brown's proof, and I have to admit that those numbers keep coming to mind as an important part of the answer. Rheumatoid arthritis is a big, big business.

I've been in treatment with Dr. Brown for the past four years. The pain has disappeared, my spirits have risen, and the swelling that threatened to put me in a wheelchair is now so minor and infrequent that I have no sign of it for as long as a year at a time. I have started my own company in the computer business, something I could never have done in my previous condition.

I wasn't the only one to make a career change. Before the agreed-upon six months were up, I got a letter from my original doctor. It said an opportunity had come along and he was moving to another city. I have since learned that he is no longer practicing as a rheumatologist, and is now a pediatrician.

CHAPTER 14

Connective Tissue

Connective tissue makes up one-third of our body weight, most of it in the form of collagen, which is the protein substance of the white fibers of skin, tendon, bone, cartilage, and nails. Collagen plays an extremely important role in the life of our joints. It is the principal component of the synovium and the plasticlike cartilaginous pads at the ends of our bones that protect the skeleton from grinding itself to powder. And it is the stuff arthritis feeds on.

For the student of arthritis, collagen has some other interesting properties—and in some important respects it is similar to its enemy, the mycoplasmas. You can see the most dramatic of those similarities if you remove the collagen from the skin of a pig. The most likely way for you to extract it is in a form that looks like cotton, in long, fibrous strands. If you put that cottony substance in a test tube and dissolve it with dilute hydrochloric acid, it goes into a solution. Next, put the solution through a filter that withholds all cells. What you now have is a filtrate that looks like pure water and, considering how it was made, would seem to be as free of living matter. But all you have to do is add a touch of table salt to recreate the long, fibrous strands of its original form.

Because this procedure has filtered out all cells, we know that the reconstituted fibers cannot be living matter. What we have instead is a natural plastic that can come and go; like mycoplasmas, collagen can change its state, traveling in and out of the visible world.

COLLAGEN AND AGING

When people get old, the reason they become wrinkled is that the connective tissue between the cells is washed out and the absence of the collagen creates furrows, like mountains and valleys.

When people get rheumatoid arthritis, they appear to age in this same way, but prematurely. The reason is the same, although with arthritis the collagen between the cells is washed out artificially by the active inflammatory process.

Some years ago I read that Colonel Earl Ashe, head of the Armed Forces Institute of Pathology and one of the country's great physicians, had given a speech in Texas in which he said that the cells of the body are immortal, and that the aging process is due to changes in the connective tissue. It was a good line, one that used hyperbole to make an important point. I ran into Ashe some months later at a medical meeting, and I congratulated him on what I had read. He knew that my whole career had focused on connective tissue—what makes it weak and what allows it to become strong again. He smiled when I shook his hand. "I thought of you when I said it," he said. "I knew you'd like it."

If physicians and researchers can find a way to turn off the process that keeps the collagen weak, it will become strong very quickly. The arthritic process keeps the collagen bathed in toxic substances, much in the same way that flame under a test tube can keep the contents unnaturally hot. If the heat is taken away, nature automatically regenerates that connective tissue. People with rheumatoid arthritis always look older than they really are. When they go into remission, the connective tissue begins to regenerate and fill up the gaps, so they automatically look years younger. And they feel a lot younger, too.

TOXINS AND TISSUE

If you look at the thighs of patients whose knees are inflamed with arthritis, the muscles appear thin and wasted and the patient has difficulty rising from a chair or going up and down stairs. The reason for this condition is the same in the muscles and skin as in the joints: the toxic substances generated in inflamed tissues in the knee run up the leg through the lymphatic system and in the process weaken the connective tissues, primarily the collagen supporting the muscle cells. The muscle fibers themselves are not affected, and when the knee inflammation is arrested the collagen re-forms and the muscle strength returns. Only if the cause of the inflammation in the joints can be reached and the inflammatory toxins arrested does the collagen have a chance to regenerate. The muscle fibers automatically fill out because a lot of the thinness is due to the loss of connective tissue. Even more importantly, the muscles begin to work again at what an engineer would call their design levels, as the supporting structure of the connective tissues is gradually restored.

Rheumatoid arthritis is a problem of the connective tissues. The inflammatory reaction—where the antibody and the antigen meet—takes place within those tissues and nowhere else. The antigen originates from the mycoplasma and comes out of a cell or on a cell, and the antibody circulates around the system until they clash on this one battleground, producing the toxicity (the formation of proteolytic enzymes) that is so damaging to those tissues.

And what is the substance of those toxins? It can be a mixture of a number of different components: proteolytic enzymes, perhaps a little histamine (an allergy-producing substance), kinins, kallikreins—a whole variety of irritants.

The clash between antigen and antibody in rheumatoid arthritis is the same as the conflict that occurs when you have a runny nose from hay fever or irritated bronchials that constrict from asthmatic allergies; a similar substance is released, causing the observed reaction.

In the case of arthritis, the release of those toxins is damaging, but the damage is not necessarily permanent. If the collagen weakness remains unabated, the body senses that the afflicted tissues might lose their structural integrity and split apart. For that reason, nature reinforces the silk of collagen with the burlap of scar tissues, accounting for the nodules and scarlike swellings in areas of marked inflammation. In cases where the inflammation burns out completely, much of that scar tissue will be absorbed and replaced once again by collagen.

CHAPTER 15.

Symptoms and Diagnosis

For the victim of rheumatoid arthritis, tangible evidence of the disease may not show up in a form that can be readily identified until it reaches its acute stage, with nodules at the joints and even disfigurement. But the physician who sees the patient in time can recognize the first symptoms far earlier, perhaps as much as a year and a half before these external physical changes occur.

WHAT DOCTORS TELL PATIENTS

The first sign of rheumatoid arthritis is not pain, but fatigue with no good reason. The history of the fatigue and of what the patient does about it often follows a predictable pattern. As a rule, when the victim realizes that he or she needs more and more sleep, the logical response is to see a family practitioner. Several tests are done, and the doctor usually reports that there is no apparent physical cause for the condition. He then asks the patient, "What's bothering you? You seem to be under a great deal of tension."

The physician is on pretty safe ground. Every person who ever visited a doctor is under some kind of stress; that's the nature of modern living. The patient thinks about it for a moment, and then acknowledges that the doctor is right. In this brief exchange, for no other reason than that the doctor can't figure out what's wrong, some of the responsibility for the symptoms has been subtly shifted to the patient. The doctor nods in affirmation and says, "Well, you'll be all right. I think that's all it is."

One of the other symptoms of rheumatoid arthritis is depression. That takes a lot of the fight out of a person, so at this point, many patients meekly get up and go home. Others are unwilling to be dismissed that quickly, and they ask the doctor if there's anything he can do to make them feel better and restore their former energy. Sometimes the physician prescribes shots of vitamins, but as a rule he says no, that things will get better by themselves.

The next step, before there is any visible change, can be an unexplained anemia. This is something a little more tangible for the doctor, who now tells the patient he knows the cause of the problem and sets about curing it with shots of vitamin B-12, iron, and sometimes folic acid.

But the hemoglobin doesn't rise as it should, and the doctor asks the patient more questions: "Are you taking the medication I've given you?" and "Is there something you're not telling me?" The patient says yes to the first and no to the second, but the questions have served a secondary purpose: the seeds of uncertainty have been planted, and the patient wonders if the real root of the problem is something he is doing that he shouldn't, or not doing that he should.

Another preliminary symptom of rheumatoid arthritis can be unexplained weight change, and this takes two forms. In some cases, people who are slight of build will lose weight; when accompanied by severe fatigue this is often a precursor of the painful phase of the disease. In other cases, the patient is already overweight, and as the disease progresses the patient's weight increases, despite efforts to control it. We have observed this same phenomenon of weight abnormality in patients with other connective-tissue diseases, including scleroderma and lupus. But as any of these diseases go into remission, both extremes begin to move nearer to the mean; patients who are too thin start to gain, and those who are obese find that their efforts to reduce are becoming more productive.

ALTERNATIVE DIAGNOSES

It usually isn't long after these various symptoms appear before the patient begins to get some joint pain. There is still no visible external evidence of change, but the pain is a new symptom and calls for another trip to the doctor. At this stage, and even as long as a year later when the pain combines with some of the early signs of disfigurement, many doctors are still unwilling to diagnose the condition as arthritis. Favorite alternatives are sciatica, bursitis, lumbago, and synovitis; the apparent rationale is that any curable disorder is preferable to one that is not.

By the same token, if the doctor understands that rheumatoid arthritis can indeed be cured, then he also recognizes that all of these delays are detrimental to the patient and can greatly extend the degree and duration of treatment.

PROVING THE PRESENCE OF THE ARTHRITIC INFECTION

If a patient comes to me with the earliest of these symptoms and nothing external yet shows, I start off with a test for the mycoplasma complement fixing reaction. It was through this means that I recently confirmed my suspicions about the eleven-year-old daughter of a woman I had been treating for several years.

The daughter was always tired and wasn't doing well in

school, and I suspected a combination of fatigue and depression, the classic early signs of rheumatoid arthritis. Like most children, she was unwilling to admit to much of anything that would aid in her diagnosis. This was partly because of a natural tendency for children to hide their feelings from adults as they seek to establish their own identities, and partly because of a lack of experience against which to make useful comparisons about how they *should* feel. Depression is particularly hard for adolescents to handle or for doctors to recognize; it doesn't show in children the way it does in adults, and is mixed in with a lot of psychological and physical changes that are normal parts of growing up. As a rule, it manifests itself as indifference. The child doesn't get out and play with others of the same age but is more inclined to read, watch television, or simply withdraw.

Despite the mother's insistence that her daughter probably had arthritis, because that was the way her own had begun when she was more or less the same age, the girl's doctors were not inclined to accept a lay diagnosis, especially when their own standard tests for the disease were negative. But when a sample of her blood was sent to our laboratory, the far more sensitive mycoplasma complement fixing reaction showed a high degree of activity, and I immediately wrote to her mother that the test, combined with the girl's other symptoms and her history, gave strong evidence of rheumatoid arthritis infection. We started her on a course of antibiotic therapy, and because it was still relatively early in the course of the disease, she picked right up and did very well.

At the end of the summer, however, my young patient hit a slump. Her spirits dropped again and she showed some of the earlier lethargy, though not as strongly. Her parents were prepared for this to happen. The mother knew from her own long experience that there are three flare periods in early stages of the treatment for rheumatoid arthritis: September, February, and May, the months in which the barometer is least stable. At those times, a doctor has to reassure his patient that it is normal for the recovery to slow down and even lose some ground for short periods, but that the slump won't last and that as the treatment continues the dips eventually stop occurring.

Up to the time of this writing, my patient, now fourteen, has had rheumatoid arthritis for three years and has been in treatment for two. Her energy levels have risen, her symptoms of depression have vanished, she gets along on a normal amount of sleep for a girl her age, her earlier outgoing nature has returned, and her grades in school are up to honor levels.

The mycoplasma complement fixing reaction by which she was initially diagnosed is a test for the antibody that develops in the bloodstream in response to a mycoplasma infection. In order to do the test, it is necessary to have strains of mycoplasma available in the laboratory. So far, no such strains are obtainable from commercial sources, so the Arthritis Institute propagates and stocks its own supply. However, it would be a simple enough matter for a pharmaceutical manufacturer to produce such a product. As mycoplasmas finally gain recognition as the cause of rheumatoid arthritis, laboratory testing kits should soon be appearing on the market.

ARTHRITIS AND TEMPERATURE

There is one other symptom involved in rheumatoid arthritis, but it is a subtle one and easy to overlook in a diagnosis. That is a very slight temperature elevation. Lyme disease is a form of rheumatoid arthritis that in its early stages presents itself differently from other types, and a pronounced fever is one of its more dramatic features. (Lyme disease has played a key role in improving the medical community's understanding of rheumatoid arthritis as an infectious illness, and is discussed in detail in Chapter 16.) With other rheumatoid forms, the temperature is usually just a fraction above normal, and the few tenths or a single degree of abnormality will often escape detection. If the temperature is measured with an electronic thermometer, however, in a doctor's office or a hospital, the slight elevation can be seen easily. It isn't the response to an invading germ, as is the case with Lyme disease, but rather is a reaction to a substance which the germ produces. This small temperature difference is one of the most exact objective indicators of profound fatigue, and often of the depression that goes with it. Once the patient has begun treatment with an antibiotic, the temperature flattens right out at normal.

This small rise in temperature is less significant as a guide to diagnosis than it is as a further proof that rheumatoid arthritis is an infection, and it is a sensitive indicator to the effect of treatment. I often make use of it when I do patient rounds at the hospital. If I see from the chart that the small fever has disappeared, I'll tell the patient I am glad to see he or she is feeling better. It's a great trick, and until I explain it, the patients often feel I have a special diagnostic gift.

HYPERSENSITIVITY

One of the central concepts for understanding how rheumatoid arthritis works is that of the "sensitized host." Hypersensitivity is really the same thing as an allergy, but it occurs in a system where it doesn't produce a standard allergic display, such as hives or the rash from poison ivy.

The human body is made up of three sections. The ectoderm includes the skin, part of the eyes, the lungs, and part of the trachea and esophagus. The entoderm is the gastrointestinal tract and its attachments. The mesoderm includes the connective tissue, bone and cartilage, muscles, nerves, blood and blood vessels, the lymph system, and the remaining glands and organs.

Each of these sections is separate in the embryo, and although they combine in later stages of development, each retains its own unique status all through life, each reacting differently and each the target of various allergies, although the entoderm can include some ectodermal and some mesodermal features.

It has occurred to me over the years that the mesoderm is primarily the focus for bacterial allergy, while the ectoderm is more the target of chemical allergy. Obviously bacteria are chemical as well, but I am referring more to such irritants as ragweed, dust, and smoke. The distinction is not complete, because we can get hives from a vaccination or from a food reaction, but the three sections do react differently even to the same stimuli.

Mesodermal allergies don't show on the surface, and because of that we don't generally call them allergies; for that matter, for a long time we didn't even call them hypersensitivities. But as time has passed, I have become convinced that one of the major pathogenic components of rheumatoid arthritis is the fact that the mesoderm is reacting in a truly allergic sense to the agents for which it is the particular target. These agents include mycoplasma, streptococcus, brucella (the agent of undulant fever, which gives rise to arthritis), tubercle bacillus, and others.

NODULES: THE CLASSIC HARBINGER

The most pronounced and classic symptom of rheumatoid arthritis is the nodule, which appears at the joints as the first external evidence of arthritic disfigurement. Because this is so widely recognized for what it represents, some victims of the disease are actually relieved when the first rheumatoid nodule appears; now, at last, the patient has something tangible to take to the doctor. Nodules usually arise at the site of some injury, such as a sprain or bump, and although it is possible to have one or two without necessarily having arthritis, it is likely that all such nodules are the result of disease activity at the site.

Nodules are unlike malignant lesions that keep on spreading, however, and they can come and go. Sometimes a patient

will detect one on an elbow or wrist and make an appointment with the doctor, only to discover that the nodule has
receded and perhaps even disappeared by the time the
appointment is kept. Or it can vanish in one place and reap-
pear later in another.

The most likely explanation for these nodules is that they
contain fibrous tissue that forms in a skein around the small
lesions where the mycoplasmas are located. The tissue is a
protective response by the body to contain the infection and
keep it from spreading. If the mycoplasma antigen stops
coming out for some reason, either because the body's
defense puts it down for a while or a medicine suppresses it,
then the scar tissue surrounding the germ is no longer needed
and the nodule goes away. The process by which this occurs is
one of natural attrition; cells are periodically replaced, and if
the cause for defense is no longer there, the body will remove
the old cells without sending in new ones.

THE ROLE OF STREPTOCOCCUS

People who have the most rheumatoid nodules are frequently the ones who have had a streptococcal infection, perhaps in childhood, and in whom there is evidence that the
streptococcal antibodies are still present along with the mycoplasmas. The drugs for streptococci are not the same as the
ones used for mycoplasmas. If I detect streptococcal antibodies, I will combine an antistreptococcal approach with the
treatment for the mycoplasma at the outset, and once the
streptococcal level has been lowered, I will focus the attack
more precisely on the mycoplasma.

The standard treatment for streptococcus is penicillin or
one of its many derivatives. Penicillin has no value in treating
the forms of rheumatoid arthritis that are caused by
mycoplasmas—the vast majority of such cases. (They do work
on the form known as Lyme disease, however, which evidence indicates is caused by a spirochete bacterium.) Con-

versely, the tetracyclines aren't as effective as penicillin in treating streptococcal infections. The problem in using penicillin-based antibiotics is that they tend to create drug allergies after a certain amount of time, so there is an incentive to limit the duration of their use. After a short term of treatment with penicillin derivatives, the rheumatoid nodules tend to disappear in patients who have the history of streptococcal infection.

HOW RHEUMATOID ARTHRITIS WORKS: A CONCEPTUAL VIEW

There are lots of other variables that have to be considered in assessing a patient's condition and monitoring the effectiveness of treatment. Most of them are subtle and some are highly elusive. But all of them have in common that they are totally incompatible with the methodology of double-blind controls, which up to now has been the universal technique by which treatments for rheumatoid arthritis are evaluated. Even the smallest of these added factors calls into doubt the reliability of the results achieved in treating the basic disease.

Over the course of the half-century in which I have studied rheumatoid arthritis, bit by tiny bit I have developed a medical design based on a conceptual view of how rheumatoid arthritis works. That view is extremely important in the decisions I make about the basic approach to treatment and in the fine tuning as that treatment progresses. In my mind, I constantly see what is going on inside a patient's body, much as I suppose atomic physicists envision the mostly invisible electrons and protons with which they work. Any physician who treats rheumatoid arthritis must develop this same conceptual view of the mechanism as a frame of reference for the process he is managing, both in formulating short-term tactical responses and in designing an overall strategy for each patient.

OTHER TESTS

The mycoplasma complement fixing reaction is just one of several tests I order when I am seeing a patient for the first time. I also routinely ask for a complete blood test which measures the hemoglobin, red blood count, white blood count, differential white cells, and other factors. White blood cells, which are the body's first line of defense against disease, are divided into several types: lymphocytes, monocytes, granulocytes, basophils, and so on. These differential white cells can shift when under attack, and if rheumatoid disease is very active the lymphocytes go up.

That rise in lymphatic activity is an excellent gauge of the progress of treatment for rheumatoid arthritis. But long before I took advantage of that useful feature, I became interested in lymphocytes for another reason: they increase during rheumatoid activity, and the polymorphonuclear cells do not. Polymorphonuclear cells are the ones that increase during appendicitis, lobar pneumonia, or staphylococcal or streptococcal infections, for example, because it is their job to go after regular bacteria that invade the body. Lymphocytes are quite different; for the most part, their tasks are related to the immune system, particularly the creation of gamma globulins. They are activated by viruses of all kinds. They are also activated by the cousins of the viruses—the mycoplasmas—against which they generate antibodies.

When I first observed this phenomenon many years ago, I began to look at diseases other than arthritis in which the lymphocytes were high. I saw that they were also very elevated in rheumatic fever, as well as in a great many other rheumatic-type illnesses such as lupus and scleroderma. I began to monitor their levels during treatment of patients with tetracycline in order to confirm that the lymphocytes were indeed performing the role I envisioned. Those studies showed such an exact cause-and-effect relationship that I now use the same tests as a barometer of the patients' progress toward recovery. If the physician wants to get a quick preview of what the laboratory technician will see under the microscope, all he has to do is touch the lymph nodes in the patient's neck; swollen glands indicate high lymphocyte activity.

Sedimentation

Another simple blood test that tells the physician a lot is the sedimentation rate. It was found long ago that when blood is put in a tube with an anticlotting substance, the cells settle to the bottom of the tube in a predictable and diagnostically useful fashion, a reversal of the way cream rises as it separates from milk. A line forms in the tube. Above that line is the straw-colored component of blood which is the plasma, and at the bottom are the red cells. The line itself, a thin layer just above the sinking bottom portion, is made up of the white blood cells. The speed at which these cells settle out of solution correlates with the rate of activity of the rheumatoid process—how "hot" it is.

The doctor or technician measures the distance the blood settles in the tube in one hour. Sedimentation rates vary by gender: a rate of 30 or below is normal for a woman, and 15 for a man. The reason for this 100 percent difference is probably related in part to the fact that the blood sedimentation rate rises when a woman menstruates. Typically, with active rheumatism the readings will be ten points higher than normal in either sex. Sedimentation testing is not entirely specific for arthritis—any inflammatory reaction will produce the same results—but it provides a good diagnostic indicator and it is also useful in monitoring the effectiveness of treatment if given every six months or so.

Bentonite Flocculation

Every incoming patient is also given a Bentonite flocculation test and a latex fixation test. Both use foreign substances that react with certain globulins that produce a kind of anti-antibody called the rheumatoid factor. This anti-antibody is a second line of defense for the body in fighting off the arthritis infection; when it tests positive the condition is more dangerous and more difficult to treat because it means the source of antigen is surrounded more vigorously by an additional wall of defending substances. The tests vary in that Bentonite flocculation is more delicate and will often give positive results when the latex test is still negative. Bentonite is also sensitive to other infections and allergies, however, while the latex test is more specific to rheumatoid arthritis. A second reason we give them both is that by the time the reaction shows positive on latex as well, we have one more clue to how far the disease has developed.

SMAC

Another standard requirement when I accept a new patient is the SMAC (for Sequential Multiple Analyzer Computer), a total blood appraisal including different chemical tests. Alkaline phosphotase, for example, if way out of line, indicates that the liver isn't just right, and creatinine, a waste product excreted only in the urine, provides clues to kidney function. Cholesterol and triglycerides are also tested. The SMAC also shows albumin levels of the blood, which are depressed if arthritis is very active and come back up to normal as the patient gets better. Other chemicals that change in the presence of arthritic activity are calcium, phosphorus, sodium, potassium, and uric acid; some go higher and some lower.

In addition to being comprehensive, the SMAC is also very accurate because it is automated. This is a distinct advantage over human measurement of these same minute quantities, a procedure which varies widely from lab to lab and from test to test, even on the same source. The SMAC makes it possible to compare test results obtained on opposite coasts, which previously would have been nearly meaningless.

The importance of accuracy and reproducibility in such tests can be seen in an exercise I did some years ago in connection with uric acid. At certain levels uric acid is associated with gout, which is easily confused with rheumatoid arthritis. When I was at George Washington University, because I was very skeptical about the reliability of manual testing, I sent a blood sample from one person to four different laboratories for a uric acid determination—and I got back four entirely different results. In one case the reading was a clear indication of gout. In another, it showed the patient was entirely free of it. The automation of these tests is a great step forward; without reproducibility, their results would be worthless.

Joint Scan

If the patient is admitted to the hospital, the next diagnostic procedure is a joint scan, using a gamma camera to view the way in which technetium 99, a rapidly degradable radiopharmaceutical, concentrates in the affected areas. The so-called "hot spots" where the concentration is heaviest provide a graphic, dynamic, and objective measure of the degree of arthritic activity of the joints. When viewed in sequence over the course of a prolonged treatment, two or three annual scans also make good visual reports on the progress of therapy, a feature that is as uplifting to the patient as it is informative to the doctor.

Kunkle Test

Another standard diagnostic procedure is the Kunkle test, a special gamma globulin measurement of how hard the body is fighting against the mycoplasma. Gamma globulin is a combined globulin that is the precursor of certain types of specific antibodies in the blood. If a person is suffering from typhoid fever, for example, the body calls on the gamma globulin pool to make antibodies against the typhoid germ. If somebody in the household has hepatitis and we want to avoid getting it, we will go to the doctor for a shot of gamma globulin because it contains a number of different antibodies that have built up in the donor's body over the years, including, possibly, some antibodies to hepatitis.

X Rays in Diagnosis

As a final diagnostic tool, if they seem to be indicated, I also order X rays. The principal area in which X rays are helpful is the hips, which are different from most of the other parts of the body in the ways they react to rheumatoid arthritis. Hips can become badly damaged even when the rest of the body is improving. This is largely because of the way they are formed and connected to their arteries. The circulation in the hip is different from that in the femur in the legs; it comes through the socket of the hip into the head and down to the neck. The shaft of the femur, on the other hand, is circulated by vessels that go down the side of the leg and then into the bone. People who are very active physically and who are likely to damage their hips, such as dancers or high hurdlers, are also likely to damage the circulation of the head or femur, especially in cases of dislocation. If that happens, the femur shows signs of dysfunction when the rest of the leg is fine, because the socket of the femur doesn't necessarily conform with the state of affairs that pertains to rheumatoid activity. It is hard to know whether this circulatory liability is also a part of the pathology of arthritis. But whether it is or not, the problem is not nearly as serious today as it was a few years ago, thanks to advances in hip prosthetic technology and new surgical techniques.

The primary purpose of all these tests, beyond aiding in the diagnosis, is the establishment of a baseline. It is also worth mentioning that the purpose of the blood tests we order during the course of treatment differs from the purpose of such tests in virtually all other forms of rheumatoid arthritis therapy: we are measuring the effectiveness of our treatment in curing the disease, not how quickly the patient is being poisoned by his or her medicine.

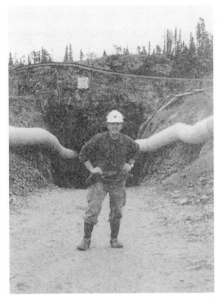

Thomas Schuster, Vancouver, Canada, age 29, Reiter's syndrome diagnosed 1994.

I could no longer stand without a cane and was contemplating life in a wheelchair. Just fifteen months after starting antibiotic therapy, there are still days when I have to take it easy, but now I am actively pursuing my career as a geologist, biking a fair amount and even starting to rock climb again.

Bob Murphy, Boynton Beach Fla. Bob's career as a professional golfer nearly ended with a diagnosis of psoriatic arthritis.

I decided to pursue the antibiotic treatment following a conversation with a friend who has rheumatoid arthritis. My sed rate was 35 on my initial visit; it fell to 3 in one year. I am proud to return to the PGA Senior Tour after four years on the sidelines, and I constantly recommend this therapy to others.

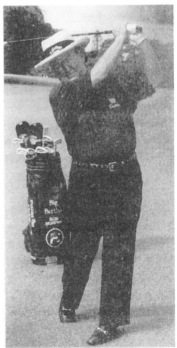

157

CHAPTER 16

Depression and Other Psychological Parameters

The organic aspect of rheumatoid arthritis—the deformity, crippling, and pain—is obvious to everybody. When psychological problems appear, as they inevitably do, many physicians regard them as a forerunner of the disease or an aspect of stress that would be natural with any chronic, progressive problem. It has not been generally recognized that these psychological symptoms are actually a component of the disease process itself.

"IT'S ALL IN YOUR HEAD"

When patients go to a doctor for treatment of their arthritis, they seldom mention these psychological problems. In some cases, the patients don't believe they are related to the disease. In other cases, the patients are afraid the doctor will think the psychological symptoms are causative and will request that the patient seek psychiatric care before undertaking the treatment of the disease. These patients are used to being told that the problem is "all in the head," and they don't want to add any more fuel to the fire. Many arthritis patients have sought psychiatric care but found that it did not help their arthritis, despite some mental relief. We have found at the Arthritis Institute that the psychological symptoms of arthritis are indeed a component of the disease process, and when the disease goes into remission, these symptoms clear up. Of all the aspects of successful treatment for which the patient is grateful, by far the most important is relief of the psychological problems which are a part of the disease. Despite their importance, however, they are the least recognized by friends, family members, associates and physicians. Severely depressed rheumatoid arthritics have long since stopped talking about their disease because they know that nobody wants to hear about it, including their doctors, so they live with it inside of them, and the pressure of suppression only makes things worse. What the patients feel when those psychological symptoms finally depart is enormous relief and gratitude.

As noted, there are a number of psychological or invisible physical symptoms that usually precede the development of the rheumatoid disease expressions by a year or longer. When confronted with the characteristic unexplained fatigue, the doctor's first suspicion is of anemia or low thyroid function. Usually all tests prove to be negative at this point. If anemia does exist, it is not generally corrected by simple measures.

Other such symptoms are an inability to concentrate as well as usual and a loss of interest in avocations and hobbies that were previously sources of enjoyment. The short-fuse syndrome is very common in this phase, and in many patients who are ordinarily very calm and well controlled it is totally alien to their normal personalities. The annoyances that the patient expresses are usually justified, but not to the degree the patient exhibits. After a particularly energetic outburst, the patient is usually chagrined, but only when it seems too late to easily correct it.

DEPRESSION IS ORGANIC

By far the most disturbing of any of the psychological symptoms is depression. Generally it comes in very short episodes, lasting from just a few hours to a few days. When the depression hits, it can be devastatingly severe, but is seldom suicidal. In the more than forty years I've been observing the behavior patterns of the rheumatoid arthritic patient, I've known of only two who committed suicide at the height of one of these depressive episodes; both were in psychotherapy at the time of death.

A FAMILY DISEASE

Family members, like doctors, usually attribute the arthritic's depression to the pain and distress that go along with the disease process, and they don't recognize it as a symptom in its own right. Those in close contact with such patients urge them to go out and do something different, to become active, and this only aggravates the situation. As these episodes of depression are generally short, it is far better to leave the patient alone until the condition passes.

It is extremely important for family and close friends to recognize the nature of this depression and that it is a part of the disease. In that respect and in many others, arthritis is a family disorder; this recognition is the best treatment the patient can possibly receive, and it is equally healing to those who give it.

Even in intimate family life, however, those who live with the patients are seldom able to share fully in the feelings of the arthritic or to help through the standard methods of encouragement. At the National Hospital, the first thing many new patients experience is a feeling of tremendous relief at being able to talk about their arthritis with those in the beds around them, people who are interested and who share their experience. People have a great need to express themselves about things that weigh heavily on their lives and to prove to themselves that their afflictions are not unique. They also need to learn that people actually get better, that they are able to recover from a disease that everyone else has told them is supposed to go progressively downhill. Husbands or wives of arthritics are victims of this same depression, only at second hand. They are constantly trying to cheer up their mates, trying to coax them into some kind of activity that will take them out of themselves, and they are constantly being thwarted by a mate who is often too depressed to move. I have had many patients over the years whose marriages have held together only because the time was taken to carefully explain the role of depression and how it can affect relationships. And I have had many others whose marriages had already ended.

PARTNERS

There are two kinds of partners of rheumatoid arthritics. One type of husband is very supportive of his wife and will do anything for her—and instinctively leaves her alone when she's depressed, not trying to jolly her out of it, because he knows it doesn't work. He watches for the moments when the sun begins to shine and then takes her out to enjoy it. Arthritics have sudden ups and downs, either with pain, fatigue, depression, or other psychological symptoms, and the mate must learn how to take advantage of the highs without becoming ensnared in the lows.

The other type of mate fights the disease, and part of that fight takes the form of denial. Arthritics are truly not responsible for the mood swings created by their affliction any more than they are responsible for the pain and crippling. Depression will not go away simply by willing it to stop.

Families need a great deal of help in understanding and coping with the disease. The majority of the patients who have these multitudinous problems look quite well, and they are unable or unwilling to say how they really feel, knowing full well that others don't want to hear discouraging things. Besides, to discuss how you hurt is boring to others. The psychological difficulties associated with arthritis are thought to be caused by an immunologic defect, and not by a personality flaw in the patient. Learning the proper response to a depression which has this organic base does not necessarily require the skills of a psychiatrist; it is mostly a matter of common sense. It is a great step forward when the patient learns that his psychological behavior pattern is part of the disease process itself and that it will improve when the cause of the disease is recognized and treated—and that it will not improve in any lasting way when symptoms alone are treated.

STRESS-PROOFING THE ARTHRITIC

An important step the treatment of any rheumatic or collagen vascular disease problem is the removal of any unnecessary stress. It is useful for the husband and wife to appear together for the interview with the doctor and to tape the conversation for further reference and understanding at later stages in the course of treatment. Rheumatoid arthritis is complicated and its treatment embraces some elusive concepts which are often particularly difficult to retain when the patient's memory is below par as a result of the disease. One of the concepts which the patient should hear and record is that long-term treatment of the basic problem will restore the memory to normal functioning.

After all these years of treating rheumatoid arthritis, I am convinced that the most important aspect of the disease is, surprisingly, not the pain but the way a person feels about himself. The lifting of depression and the regaining of interest, the desire for accomplishment, the improved mental functioning, all seem to give the patient a new life. The process of premature aging comes to an end and the patient realizes there is a great deal left to live for.

There could be no understanding of the relationship

between the psychological parameters and the disease process itself until it was possible to reach the source of the problem. It seems clear from our experience that the basic problem is not addressed by any of the symptomatic treatments. On the contrary: In the long run, the traditional treatment methods allow the fundamental disease process to progress under the cover of symptomatic relief.

We have also found that psychological parameters are of vital importance in determining the distance covered on the road back. These psychological factors have not been generally recognized or employed as they should be, as important milestones for measuring and marking therapeutic accomplishment.

CHAPTER 17

John Doe, M.D.: The Doctor as Patient

This case history has been disguised at the subject's request. Dr. Doe, a gerontologist, lives and practices in a Virginia suburb of Washington, D.C.

I had my first symptoms of rheumatoid arthritis in the fall of 1984. They began as neck pains, and at first I suspected the cause was the position of my head on the pillow during sleep. Although they were worst in the mornings, they pretty well disappeared after an hour or two, and there were some days when I didn't have any pains at all. But after they had persisted intermittently for about a month, I went to my family doctor for a test of my RA factor. (The RA, or rheumatoid factor, is a relatively recent discovery and has proven to be very valuable in the diagnosis of rheumatoid disease.) The result was positive, and he sent me to a rheumatologist.

By the time I kept that second appointment another two weeks had passed, and the pain had spread to my right shoulder. Part of my practice as a physician involves physical exertion in dealing with elderly patients, and I found the condition was beginning to interfere with my ability to help them on and off the table and to assist them in changing positions during examinations. However, I saw the rheumatologist in the afternoon at a time when my pain wasn't bothering me, and he said to me, "Well, Doctor, you look just fine," and gave me a prescription for ibuprofen, an anti-inflammatory analgesic which had already been prescribed by my family physician.

A week later my shoulder and neck bothered me so badly I called the rheumatologist again. His answering service told me he had gone on vacation, and I left my name for the doctor who was taking his cases; that doctor, who knew nothing about me, didn't bother to return my call for three days, and by then I was in agony. When he finally did call, I told him I had gone elsewhere.

Elsewhere was a rheumatologist in Baltimore, referred by another physician from the hospital in northern Virginia with which I affiliate. I told the Baltimore doctor the case was an emergency, because the condition was now making it difficult, and at times impossible, for me to continue my practice. He was so busy he couldn't fit me in until the middle of December, more than a month away, but that was a lot better than being out of town or not returning my call, so we set a date.

At our first meeting he said he wanted to admit me to the Baltimore hospital for further study, and I agreed to a week in early January 1985. I was reluctant, because it meant taking time off from work at my own hospital and required the re-scheduling of a lot of my elderly patients who do not take well to change.

By the time I entered the hospital, the pain in my neck had improved noticeably. My shoulder was worse, and there were new pains in one knee and the opposite hip. The study involved a joint survey with whole-body X rays and a full repeat of all the laboratory tests I had undergone earlier. While I was going through this, I noticed that I was beginning to feel light-headed and slightly dizzy, and all my joints were starting to get unusually warm, which I mentioned to the doctor. He wasn't surprised; he told me the tests showed my hemoglobin had dropped from my normal of 12 or 13 to 10 grams and the sedimentation rate was up 20 points to 55. He took my temperature rectally and it stayed normal; only my joints were hot. When the tests were completed, I was sent home with three prescriptions: one for prednisone, one for Plaquenil, and one for a nonsteroidal anti-inflammatory. My life as an arthritic had begun in earnest.

In the months that followed, I never had any fear that I would die from the arthritis, but there were many times when I seriously wondered if I would survive the treatment.

My first problem with medication was a rash which developed all over my body within two weeks of leaving the hospital in Baltimore. I called for a return appointment, but the problem with seeing a successful rheumatologist between regular visits is that the patient has to sit for up to five hours in the waiting room surrounded by chronic-looking patients, and each such journey turns into a day-long expedition. Already, I had sacrificed more of my professional time to the treatment than to the disease itself, and the situation was only to get worse in the months ahead. When the doctor finally saw me, he stopped the first nonsteroidal anti-inflammatory and put me on low levels of another one called Feldene.

Over the next few months, my life was reduced to little more than working, eating, and sleeping. I was recently divorced at the time, and a woman cousin who lives nearby in Maryland often helped with my cooking and drove me back and forth to my appointments in Baltimore. I managed to get to work on my own, but there were days when my wrists were so painful and my hands so weak I was unable to hold the steering wheel of my car and was forced to call in sick. Over the next four months, because of the steroids, my weight increased by fifty pounds, up from a normal 170 to a very uncomfortable 220.

That June I went to work one morning, put in a normal day, and at about two in the afternoon I noticed that my hands were becoming so stiff that I had trouble using them. This was an ominous departure from my usual experience, in which all of my inflammation and stiffness had occurred in the morning, and I decided to head home as quickly as possible;

something really bad was coming, and I knew if I stayed around any longer I would have to be admitted as a patient. I was not eager to advertise my physical liabilities among my peers as I was afraid it might affect my future at the hospital. When I got to my locker I was unable to open the door and had to ask an intern for help, but then I decided things were happening too quickly for me to take the time to change and I headed out to the garage. Somehow I opened the door to my car, and as I sat behind the wheel I dropped the keys on the floor. After I finally got them into the ignition lock, it took another twenty minutes to turn them enough to get the engine started. My hands had lost almost all of their strength, especially in the rotational motion of the wrist. Driving home was no problem because the car has an automatic shift and power steering, but once I reached my house I was unable to turn the wheel enough to park in the garage, so I pulled over to the curb on the street. It took another half hour to turn off the key, and that much time again to walk up the path to my front door and into the house. Once inside, I went to the bedroom and called my cousin. "I don't know what's happening," I told her, "but you'd better get right over. I can't move."

I badly needed to relieve my bladder, but I knew I'd never make it to the bathroom on my own. I lay back on the bed and waited for my cousin.

By the time she arrived, I had been lying in one position long enough that I couldn't even turn my head. I asked her to call a good friend of mine, an orthopedic surgeon, to get the name of a rheumatologist whom he had recommended several months earlier. I also called Baltimore and talked to the resident at the hospital where my present rheumatologist practiced. I told him I was suffering a severe arthritic attack and asked what I could do. He told me I could drive to Baltimore, but even if I did there wasn't much they could do for me because my regular doctor had gone home; the best he could offer was to give me some Demerol. I decided not to go. (Since I've been sick with arthritis, I have carefully avoided any of the painkillers like Demerol or morphine because of my fear of becoming addicted; the strongest medication of that kind I ever took was Darvocet-N 100, and in two years I didn't use a hundred tablets.)

My cousin dialed the rheumatologist my friend had referred me to, in a Maryland suburb of Washington and much nearer to where I lived. He agreed to see me the next day.

The following morning I was better, but not nearly well enough to go to work or to drive to the doctor's office by myself. My cousin came back at noontime and we drove to the doctor's in her car.

This time the doctor started me off on aspirin, coated to avoid disturbing my stomach, which by now had become sensitive to almost every form of medication. The doctor tried to take me off the steroids, but every time I stopped taking them I became so stiff and inflamed that he had to start me right up again. He then tried tapering my dosage to a low level of five milligrams every day, but it took five tries and six more months before he was successful in stopping the steroids altogether; during each of those failed attempts, I'd be all right for about a week, and then I'd become so stiff again I couldn't move.

But what this new rheumatologist was taking away with one hand, he started putting right back with the other. He began a program of injecting cortisone directly into my wrist joints, and a course of treatment with gold salts. The gold was like mustard in both appearance and effects. I don't know which treatment was more painful. In a short time I noticed that my normally brown hair had started turning red from the gold injections, and I asked him with a certain amount of irony if I were eventually going to become blond. A few days later I received an even more ironical answer when I discovered that the hair on the top of my head had started to fall out.

Besides all that, the gold didn't work. After five months, the doctor decided to try yet another approach and he switched me over to penicillamine.

The penicillamine was a great relief from the gold for two reasons: it was administered orally and didn't require the painful injections, and it worked. The arthritis came under control within just a few weeks, and for the next couple of months I felt terrific. Then one morning as I was shaving I felt something odd on my upper lip, somewhat like an insect bite, and as I looked more closely I saw that I was developing a blister. Within a few days it had spread to the inside of my mouth and cracked down the middle both inside and out; then it started to bleed, and pus appeared at the edges of the lesion.

The rheumatologist decided the blister had nothing to do with the treatment and he sent me to a dermatologist. The dermatologist took one look and quickly agreed; he said the blister was more likely related to the arthritis itself, and he gave me a steroid cream to spread over the affected area. By this time I was becoming certain that the real cause was the penicillamine, but when I suggested it a second time, the dermatologist said he would watch it for a while and if it got worse he would do a biopsy—not an answer that encouraged further discussion.

Shortly after the blister appeared, I began to notice new symptoms in my eyes. I had always been highly allergic by nature, reacting to almost everything from dust to feathers to pollen and all the other known irritants, and as a result I was not unused to having my eyes become red and teary. But this was something new; whenever the reaction started, it would come on like a tornado and I would be nearly blinded by the water in my eyes. I wondered whether it might be stress-related, but I dismissed that idea when I considered that my arthritis was better than ever, I was able to do my job well enough, and my life seemed to be relatively stress-free.

I went to see an eye doctor who told me it was probably just an unusual form of allergy. He gave me some drops to put in several times a day. One morning a week later I looked in the bathroom mirror, and what I saw there belonged in a Dracula movie; my eyes were fiery red. The ophthalmologist didn't have any new ideas and just told me to continue using the drops. But a few days after that I was at work and I ran into an eye surgeon who took one look at me and asked if I had rheumatoid arthritis. When I said I did, he examined my eyes closely and told me that my tear ducts had stopped producing tears, a not-uncommon effect of the disease. He gave me artificial tears, which I applied three times a day.

Meanwhile, I was developing a reaction to the aspirin which the doctor had prescribed in place of the steroids. I experienced dizziness, ringing in my ears, and light-headedness. The doctor told me to cut down, and after I did I called him back and said I planned to get off the penicillamine as well. I reasoned that if the relatively minor problems with the aspirin were sufficient to cut back, then the far more serious effects of penicillamine were a good argument for quitting altogether.

About two months later I went back for a check-up and found that all the test results had started climbing again. The penicillamine hadn't changed anything; it had merely masked the effects of the arthritis, and now they were coming back to the surface. The doctor told me he wanted to put me back on the penicillamine. I was scared to death of it but, like him, I couldn't see any other choice. I took one tablet, and the next day my lips were completely covered with blisters.

It happened that on that same day, I had my weekly appointment with the physical therapist who had been helping me to work with my affected joints. He took one look at me and said, "You know, you really ought to be seeing Dr. Brown at the National Hospital."

I had never heard of Dr. Brown, and I asked the therapist who he was. He told me about Dr. Brown's treatment, which he said was sometimes described by others as "unconventional and unproven." He said that although they had never met, he saw many of Dr. Brown's patients who were recovering from rheumatoid arthritis, and he was very impressed with the fact that they were all getting better. Without much hope for the results, I called the National Hospital for an appointment and was told Dr. Brown wouldn't be able to see me for six months. I asked the appointment secretary to put me down for the first opening, in June.

I returned to the doctor who had started me back on the penicillamine, and when he saw the new blisters he immediately switched me over to methotrexate. "This is my last one," he said. "Let's hope it works."

"Let's," I said.

I stayed on the methotrexate for four months, but when I saw Dr. Brown I stopped and have been on a simple antibiotic ever since.

Dr. Brown warned me of the Herxheimer effect when I began the tetracycline therapy, and although the effect lasted a month I could feel myself becoming better even within the first week. (The Herxheimer effect, described in Chapters 16 and 18, is a reaction to treatment in which the symptoms of a disease get worse at the start of therapy, a paradoxical sign that the infectious source of a disease is under attack.) It was as though I could actually feel what was happening at the cellular level in my body, that the cause of the arthritis was being attacked and destroyed and carried out of my system, and it was terrific.

I have been in treatment with Dr. Brown for only three months, and I have improved immensely. My hips and knees are now in perfect shape and I can walk briskly for the first time in two years; I have more energy, I can exercise more each day, my damaged hepatic function has improved, my eyes are better, and I am returning to health. The wrist joints in both arms were already damaged by the disease before I reached Dr. Brown, however, and this treatment is not going to increase their limited function. I still have a distance to go, but I feel that I am on the road to full recovery.

I wish I had heard of Dr. Brown's treatment two years earlier, in time to save me the unnecessary suffering, the expense, and the damage to my career and my body which I have lived through in the interim. And I hope by telling my small part of Dr. Brown's story, I will help the world to get to know him better and save others from my own all-too-common experience.

CHAPTER 18

Arthritis Research: A Brief Overview

Many years ago, particularly around the turn of the century, rheumatoid arthritis was generally considered to be an infectious problem. The reason for this view was that there were a certain number of people who first had kidney trouble, a bad tonsil, or some other infectious complaint and developed arthritis soon afterward. It was assumed that the focal infection was the cause of the arthritis, and that if the focus were excised, the infection would go with it.

FIGHTING INFECTION WITH SURGERY

It was an era in which surgeons moved very quickly to take out all the removable parts that could be a source of infection, such as tonsils, the appendix, ovaries, the uterus, a kidney, the gallbladder—and often the synovial membrane from the affected joints. It was a devastating period for sufferers of arthritis because many of them were on the operating table within a day or two of complaining of the first twinge in a joint. The surgery did have an impact on the arthritic condition. Some patients improved markedly, but the results were not consistent, and many others got worse. As a result of unsuccessful joint surgery, some were crippled for life.

That draconian approach to arthritis quickly turned into unwarranted excess. It went on for ten or fifteen years, until finally, like each of the successive chemical treatments in the modern era, it ran its course. The principal reason for the demise of this particular approach to the disease was the rise of the American Rheumatism Association, which stood as a bulwark against unethical practices and treatments of arthritis that clearly didn't work.

Unfortunately, when this kind of surgery fell into disrepute, the infectious theory was badly weakened as well. The baby, which was perfectly healthy, was thrown out with the bath water.

In the course of many decades of studying the disease as an infection, I have developed a theory for why some arthritics were improved by the surgery. I suspect that when some people got dramatically better after the surgical removal of a localized infection—in the gallbladder, tonsil, kidney, or wherever—it was because they were still in the early stages of the arthritic infection, and their bodies had not yet had time to become violently sensitized against the bacterial antigen. Conversely, those who did not do well after surgery were the ones who had suffered from arthritis so long that they were sensitized by exposure to the bacterial toxins—toxins that had been pouring into the bloodstream for months or years. When the focal area was attacked surgically, it released yet more toxins into the system of the already sensitized host, showing up in the form of a postoperative flare.

STEROIDS AND THE ECLIPSE OF INFECTION

At about the midpoint of this century, the infectious theory went into a steep decline as the conceptual view of the arthritic mechanism took a sudden and unexpected turn. In the late 1940s, a researcher named Philip Hench at the Mayo

Clinic announced several new extracts from the adrenal cortex, work that would win him (with E. C. Kendall and Tadeus Reichstein) a well-deserved Nobel Prize. Among those extracts was a substance he called Compound E, which had a startling impact on rheumatoid arthritis. The compound soon became known throughout the world as cortisone.

Cortisone was among the most miraculous of the new wonder drugs that followed World War II. It was absolutely astonishing to see its effects on patients who had been bed-ridden with crippling, advanced rheumatoid arthritis: they were suddenly able to rise and walk again without pain.

Most of America's rheumatologists quickly decided that the natural cortisone production in the body of an arthritic patient was simply too low, much as natural insulin production is too low in the body of a diabetic. This concept of arthritis as a kind of deficiency replaced whatever was left of the infectious theory, and much of the medical world celebrated the conquest of the world's most prevalent disease— even though the deficiency thesis was unproven and the cause of the alleged deficiency was still undetermined.

In fact, I knew from my own research that the thesis was not only unproven, but its basic premise was incorrect. The question of the role played by the glands in arthritis—the adequacy of the thyroid, the ovaries, or the adrenal gland, or the other endocrines—had been investigated extensively. It was known that the adrenal gland, where cortisone is made, was no different in arthritic patients than in patients without any trace of arthritis.

Yet the paradox remained that an excessive level of cortisone—far above what was being produced normally— would make an arthritic patient feel better. Supporters of the deficiency theory amended their thesis slightly to fit the results: they decided that although arthritics did indeed produce a normal amount of cortisone in their own bodies, it was of an inferior quality. No evidence was ever given to show in what way it was inferior or that it differed in any way from the cortisone produced by people who were perfectly healthy.

On the contrary, new evidence soon appeared that placed the deficiency theory in even more serious doubt. With a true deficiency, as in hypothyroidism, for example, replacement of the missing endocrine permits the body to keep functioning indefinitely at its normal levels; patients who take daily doses of thyroid to supplement or replace the production of a damaged or missing thyroid gland lead otherwise normal lives. But with this new "cure" for arthritis, it became apparent that after a relatively short time, usually within just a few months, the extra cortisone began to lose its effectiveness.

PROBLEMS IN PARADISE

Hench's work and the results his compound at first achieved so captured the enthusiasm of the medical world that even when cortisone's effectiveness began to decline, almost nobody wanted to turn back from the new deficiency theory that its discovery had generated. Hench himself explained the failure as a problem of the kind of cortisone that was being used, and he exhorted the medical world to find a more effective type that would last indefinitely.

For the next decade, an enormous campaign of scientific research produced one steroid after another in the hope of finding such an ideal product. But after ten years of high promises followed by inevitably dismal disappointments, the great enthusiasm behind the quest for the perfect cortisone finally began to fizzle out.

A very big additional reason for the steroid fizzle was the discovery of numerous negative effects. These included stomach ulcers, high blood pressure, diabetes, and cataracts, among other things. It was observed that in many cases, prolonged and excessive use of cortisone resulted in the loss of calcium from the bones, a fact of particular concern to older patients already suffering from osteoporosis. If arthritis were really caused by a natural deficiency, we knew from our experience with hypothyroidism that the missing endocrine could be replaced for the rest of the patient's life and no such side effects would ever arise. Even with the eventual shift away from steroids, however, the deficiency concept tarried on. When Hench suggested the problems with cortisone were just with its form, I finally began to object in public. I was certain that the adverse effects arose from the cortisone itself, and not just because the compound needed some fine tuning. I believed that cortisone's anti-inflammatory properties could still serve physicians who wanted to use the drug as an adjunct to some other form of treatment; indeed, I still use low levels to help patients through the initial stages of antibiotic therapy, or in cases where earlier misuse of steroids has destroyed the patient's ability to produce the required natural amount. But I was certain that the ways in which cortisone had been used for the ten years following its discovery had produced far more serious problems than the ones it had resolved. And I was also sure, as was the rest of the medical world by then, that whatever good things cortisone seemed to do at first, the benefits didn't last.

The impact of the discovery of cortisone on arthritis research was very similar to that of the discovery of insulin, in the early 1920s, on diabetes research. Both discoveries abruptly ended nearly all ongoing efforts to find the causes of their respective diseases. Nobody seemed to care what made arthritis or diabetes happen as long as they could control the symptoms. Years later, it was discovered that it wasn't enough just to manage blood-sugar levels with insulin, that the long-term complications from diabetes, such as retinal damage, cataracts, infections, and abscesses, still occurred.

THE ROMANCE COOLS

With the cortisone honeymoon approaching its end in the early 1960s, the American Rheumatism Association began to take a more prudent view of the use of steroids in large doses, but the medical community was still a long way from suing for divorce. Cortisone was still wonderful; it was just not as wonderful as it had been in 1950, and it had to be used in a more gingerly fashion. Although it was not said explicitly, there was a tacit recognition that what had been reluctantly identified as side effects of cortisone were not side effects at all; they were normal effects, part and parcel of using steroids in large quantities. And they could be disastrous.

Ironically, the effects of excessive cortisone had been identified and spelled out in detail a number of years earlier by the great neurosurgeon Harvey Cushing. Cushing's syndrome is a condition in which the pituitary gland, which is at the base of the brain, becomes overactive. When that happens, it makes the adrenal gland overactive as well, and the result is that the body produces too much cortisone. The effects Cushing noted from the overproduction of natural cortisone include hypertension, diabetes, cataracts, ulcers, osteoporosis, and odd distribution of body fat so that the torso becomes very large while the legs and arms remain small. Diabetes, mellitus, impotence in men, and hirsutism in women were also features of the clinical pattern. Cushing never called these phenomena side effects because he knew that they weren't side effects; they were the regular effects of too much cortisone. They had been an important part of the literature for decades.

For the whole field of arthritis research, there was a very costly long-term legacy from the introduction and spectacular early success of cortisone. That success was responsible for a nearly total commitment to the study and treatment of rheumatoid arthritis as a metabolic process, at the expense of any further study of the question of a primary infectious component. It was finally found that cortisone owed its effects to the fact that it interfered in some way with the autoimmune reaction, that it made people feel remarkably better almost immediately because it blocked the body's natural defenses. When it became apparent that the benefits didn't hold up over time, the medical profession found itself in the midst of a terrible dilemma. On one side was the immense early promise that had attached to a product that may well be the most highly publicized drug in the history of medicine. On the other was the growing body of evidence that it didn't last, and that the patient could wind up worse off than when the treatment started.

That pattern—enormous early promise, followed by terrible disillusionment—was to be repeated over and over again as an endless succession of new metabolic compounds flowed from the research laboratories of America and the rest of the world. Indeed, it would characterize the course of arthritis research for most of the next thirty years.

CORTISONE IS STILL USEFUL

I recognized that cortisone had some valuable properties in the treatment of arthritis, but from the very beginning I opposed the enthusiasm for large doses of any compound that would totally block the body's immune defense system. Cortisone in those quantities was being used like a dam in a river, and I knew that the pressure would continue to build and that sooner or later the dam would break or overflow— usually with a peptic ulcer that would start to bleed, so treatment had to be stopped—and the rebound flare would create disastrous consequences for the patient. And that is exactly what happened. When the use of cortisone at these high levels finally failed, most of the medical world had subscribed too heavily to the autoimmune theory to switch back to the possibility of infection playing a role.

Meanwhile, my own group continued working in the same old direction. Even when cortisone was at its peak of popularity, before the failures had mounted into the millions, we assumed that if there were an infectious allergy from mycoplasmas or anything else, cortisone worked simply because it blocked the allergy, not because it supplanted any natural deficiency or cured a thing. Cortisone's effect on allergies had already been well established; when people suffered from very severe status asthmaticus, for example, and were practically dead with breathing problems, cortisone would stop the attack right away by blocking the allergic reaction. Because rheumatoid arthritis responded so well, at first, to this anti-allergy substance, we began to speculate that the disease involved more of an allergic reaction than anyone had previously assumed, and we began to investigate that avenue as well. In regular allergies, the main offender is histamine release. In rheumatoid hypersensitivity, histamine is present in small amounts; the main offender is a mixture of proteolytic enzymes.

Despite its failures, over the course of the following years I frequently acknowledged our debt to cortisone for the redirection it had given to scientific thought on the question of hypersensitivity or the allergic state. It became well known that when a physician used cortisone in large quantities, and especially when that use led to dramatic remission, the disease got ten times worse when the cortisone was finally stopped. This backlash wasn't just a subjective observation of patients; it was detectable in the sudden increases in rheumatoid factor, sedimentation rate, gamma globulin, and reactive proteins, in the fall in hemoglobin, and in all the other measurable indicators by which the disease is monitored.

BACK TO THE DRAWING BOARD

Once the deficiency theory had finally run its course, the medical and scientific world slowly returned to an examination of some of the alternative causes of rheumatoid arthritis. The theory is now gradually reemerging that an infection or some other form of antigen creates a reaction which in turn causes inflammation in the joints, pain, weakness, and the other classic symptoms of the disease.

One of the first places medical researchers began to look after cortisone fizzled out was toward nonsteroidal anti-inflammatories. Suddenly a flood of such drugs appeared on the market: Naprosyn, Nalfon, Tolectin, Meclomen, Clinoril, and many more. They were designed to do what cortisone did in blocking inflammation, but without the side effects. All of these compounds passed the standard six-month double-blind screening requirements of the FDA, and they were all very promising. But over the course of longer experience, sometimes only after a couple of years of clinical use by hundreds of thousands of patients, many of the old, invidious side effects inevitably reemerged, along with some new ones. Some of these drugs caused stomach troubles; others have been discovered to cause kidney damage.

The primary impetus for the eventual turning away from cortisone, as indeed from all the other standard methods of symptomatic therapy, including gold and methotrexate in more recent years, has not been the doctors; it has been the patients. A lot of doctors resist the notion that there may be some democracy in medicine, and their resistance has slowed down the shift of arthritis research back toward treatments the patient can live with. The fact is that people are not going to tolerate medication that could easily destroy their health or their lives. Patients should be brought into the process of setting directions far sooner than they are, and they should be included deliberately, not just after everything has failed.

Most doctors pay lip service to the concept that patients should have some say in their treatment, but very few are really eager to see a system in which information about how medicines work is systematically shared and becomes the primary mechanism for setting the direction of treatment and research. A doctor feels that he is blessed with profound knowledge, as indeed he is. And he has been through the mill to learn what he knows: he's suffered through incredibly hard work in four years of college, four years of medical school, and four years of hospital training. As a rule, the patient has little of this breadth of knowledge. Patients often have a particular understanding of their own disease, however, which they have acquired from extensive reading and from conversations with others who suffer from the same affliction. The patient has something else which is extremely valuable and which many doctors do not have: direct experience with the failure or success of the various medicines which the doctor prescribes. That knowledge is absolutely imperative to the process by which such products are refined and future medicines are developed.

BREACH OF PROMISE

For most rheumatoid arthritics, this long history of broken promises and misdirections has been one of the most painful aspects of their disease. And it has created a reaction: the problem of false hope has emerged as one of the most important factors in gaining a consensus and setting the agenda for arthritis research. Patients who have been told that wonderful things will happen, only to discover that the effects don't last and that they often carry a terrible price, finally reach a point where they no longer believe in anything. That one problem, more than anything else, provides the best reason for directing research toward the cause of arthritis instead of toward its symptoms. Any medicine that eliminates the source of the problem cannot fail.

One of the things we have repeatedly demonstrated with our research on mycoplasmas is that when the treatment is aimed at the primary antigen that causes the arthritis reaction, a lot of the symptomatic drugs which had previously failed to be effective will come back to life again. An attack on the antigen itself even revives the efficacy of aspirin in patients for whom aspirin had stopped relieving pain many years earlier. Many new patients ask me what I can give them to supplant their most recent painkiller because, like all the others, it has stopped working. I tell them that I'll do something even better than that; I'll continue them on the old painkiller and make it work again.

WHY SYMPTOMATIC REMEDIES FAIL

The reason all such pain medicines eventually fail when the patient is treated symptomatically is not that the patient's system is getting any weaker, but that the antigen is becoming that much more widespread. When any such medicine removes the inflammatory barrier from around the source of the antigen, it is like removing the coolant from a nuclear power core, and the eventual result is a meltdown. The inflammation is nature's way of holding the reaction in check; it happens to be a painful method, but it is the only means by which the spread of the source of the antigen is contained. The fact that aspirin and other painkillers can be made to work again after the patient has started tetracycline therapy is more than a convenience for the management of discomfort. It is one further indication that the antibiotic is attacking the problem at its source.

LIKE A BACTERIAL ALLERGY

Essentially, rheumatoid arthritis operates in the manner of a bacterial allergy, leading to collagen vascular disturbances. It is an allergic or hypersensitive state. The reaction is most intense in the connective tissue between the cells.

By itself, each of these pieces of the rheumatoid arthritis puzzle may be little more than a curiosity. But taken together, a complete picture has formed over time, and it now provides researchers with their first full portrait of the process by which rheumatoid arthritis occurs. Only with this portrait in mind can a plan for sustained control and ultimate elimination of the disease be designed.

CHAPTER 19

Curly Knowlton

Some years ago, I had a patient named Curly Knowlton. He was a great outdoorsman, and such an expert fisherman that he could put a fly on a dime at a hundred feet—a skill which he had often demonstrated at Madison Square Garden, as well as along the banks of rivers and streams all through the American and Canadian Rockies. He supported this avocation by writing for fishing magazines and running an anglers' supply company. One day, he began to have trouble with his knees. He bought an exercise bicycle to help build them up to their old tone, but the treatment seemed to make his condition worse than before. By the time someone finally put him in touch with me, he was so badly crippled that he had been confined to a wheelchair for several months and was unable to take a step without help.

I was head of medicine at George Washington University at the time, and I recognized in Curly's situation a rare opportunity to make a dramatic point with our medical students. I learned early on that, in general, medical students don't have much interest in arthritis; they dismiss the victims as people who are simply worn out, and not worth the trouble.

And it isn't just doctors. In some respects, the unspoken

popular attitude toward arthritis seems to be that it is part of a sort of natural selection process in which nature culls out the weak. Rheumatoid arthritis afflicts three times as many women as men, is seldom fatal in its own right, and is a disease which is judged falsely as an affliction of unsturdy people whose fabric is basically flawed. Worse yet, most of the people who suffer from rheumatoid arthritis have a hang-dog attitude toward themselves and their affliction; acute depression is as real a part of the pathology as the pain and crippling. Arthritics have a hard time fighting back because they don't feel they really *deserve* much better—and that attitude may be the one contagious part of the disease.

The day the demonstration began, we collected a very large group of medical students, interns, residents, and nurses, and crowded them all into the patient's room. I knew Curly well enough to call him by his nickname at that point (he didn't have a hair on his head), and I offered him the following proposition. "Curly," I said, "I want you to cooperate in a procedure here that you may find very difficult. I'm going to ask you to stay in bed for as long as it takes us to cure your arthritis. Don't get up for anything—not even to go to the bathroom. I want to be sure that you don't give your legs any exercise at all. You've been working every day to try to make them better with your exercise bicycle, but now we're going in exactly the opposite direction and you won't do anything."

"Good God," Curly said, "if I don't have some kind of activity, I'll just fall apart!" He was a wonderful foil for my intended demonstration, and I could see that his protests were producing a dramatic effect on the audience.

"Well, I want to prove something, and this is the only way I know how," I said. "What I want to prove is that in two weeks' time, without doing a single thing yourself to improve your condition, you're going to get up out of that bed and walk all the way down the hall to the nurses' desk."

"Hell," Curly said, "that's just plain impossible." He looked to his audience, apparently hoping to find a reprieve from someone in the group who felt as strongly as he did that my plan would never work. Perhaps Curly didn't fully appreciate the relationship between a head of medicine and his students in a medical school; I, too, detected a good deal of sympathy for his position from the two dozen-odd faces around the crowded room, but no such reprieve was forthcoming—in fact, no one said a word.

"What I'm doing here is putting my reputation on the line," I told Curly and the students. "And I'm not about to make a wild claim that I can't live by. If you give me the two weeks, I'll put you back on your feet."

Realizing that he didn't have a single advocate in the roomful of sympathizers, Curly laid his head back on the pillow in defeat. Finally he looked warily back at me and asked, "How are you going to do it?" He didn't seem very interested in the answer.

"I'll treat you intravenously with an antibiotic. It will put out the fire of the disease activity in your knees or at least quiet it down, and reduce the toxins that are running up your legs and weakening your muscles. Your muscles will automatically be strengthened just by the absence of the destructive activity that's going on around them, and they will do that without exercise."

I wasn't taking any risk at all, either with my reputation or with Curly's health. If he promised not to get out of bed, I knew enough about his character to be sure he'd stick with it. And I had enough experience in treating rheumatoid arthritis to be certain of obtaining the promised results. I also knew that if I hoped to teach my students anything about how tetracycline works on arthritis, I would have to firmly close the door to any possible claim that Curly had simply exercised himself back to good health.

He waved a weak hand in affirmation. "Okay, you have a deal."

I told the medical students and the others in the audience to return there in exactly two weeks, and I named the time.

For the next fourteen days, Curly was treated with intravenous doses of tetracycline, and I checked on him and his nurses several times a day to verify that he was keeping his word about the exercise. I didn't doubt him, but I wanted to make sure that nobody missed the point.

We reassembled at the designated hour, and this time I realized that there were even more people in the room than had been there two weeks before, including some physicians from the hospital staff. I stood by the head of Curly's bed and in due course I asked him if he had followed our agreement and stayed in bed the whole time.

"Yes," he said, without much enthusiasm. "I didn't get up one single time."

"And did you take any form of exercise?"

"No," he said. "How could I?"

"All right," I said. "Now let me just ask you, Curly: Do you think that without treatment there are any circumstances under which you could have gotten out of this bed and walked down to the nurses' station?"

"No," he said, his voice rising with the anger and frustration that had been building up over the past fourteen days, "and by God I don't think there is any chance at all that I can do it now, either. I came here in a wheelchair because I couldn't walk in the first place, and I've been lying here flat on my back ever since, going to seed."

"Well," I said, "try it and we'll have a chance to see."

I pulled back the covers from his bed. He swung his legs over the side and, after a moment's hesitation, stood up. One of the nurses reached out to take his arm, but I motioned for her to step aside. Some of the spectators who crowded around the doorway backed out into the corridor as Curly put one shaky leg in front of the other and started unsteadily across the room. No one in the entire company looked more astonished than Curly himself. He rounded the corner into the hallway, and a few moments later he stood triumphantly in front of the nurses' station. Then he executed a smart about-face and walked with increasing confidence and delight back to where the grand procession had begun.

Curly's arthritis was on the mend. More to the point, from

that day forward there was a whole new generation of students at George Washington University School of Medicine who decided that arthritis was worth treating after all, that there may very well be a cause that can be defined, and that there was a treatment that could actually work.

CHAPTER 20

The Case Against Double-Blind Testing

O ne of the most enduring and contentious impediments to the conquest of rheumatoid arthritis has been the lack of an effective methodology to test its various forms of treatment. What drugs work, how do they work, and for how long do they work? What are their good effects and what are their bad ones?

There are now some two thousand remedies for arthritis. Some of them are old wives' tales, some are herbs or other natural products, and many hundreds of them are the results of pharmaceutical research based on the premise that the disease is a metabolic disorder of unknown cause. The standard medicines that have already been used on a typical arthritic before I take the case represent the best and most popular of this last class of treatment. Every one of them has passed the standard six-month double-blind crossover tests used for judging pharmaceutical compounds, and every one of them is ineffective in controlling the progress of the disease.

Double-blind testing is the method in which neither the doctor nor the patient knows whether the substance being administered is a true medicine or a placebo that does nothing. The test group is divided equally, and only when the six-month trial period has elapsed is it revealed which half got the real thing. Meanwhile, each patient's progress is followed closely for reactions and for diagnostic indications of improvement or decline.

WHY THE DOUBLE-BLIND STANDARD?

The reason this method has been successful in the development of many other kinds of medicine is that the process is beyond partisan control, and the results are free of interpretive bias. Double-blind testing works just fine when the response is linear and the process being examined is completed within the six-month test period.

The reason it does not work with drugs used in the treatment of rheumatoid arthritis is that the response is not linear and the process by which the body reacts to the medicine is seldom completed within six months. The indications of how well the drug is working can reverse themselves shortly after the product has been certified as safe, and overnight the beneficial medicine can become a deadly poison. Of all the hundreds of metabolic or symptomatic drugs that have been developed against rheumatoid arthritis over the past four decades, not a single one has stayed effective and nontoxic for a period of five years. And it is not uncommon for patients who have taken part in a double-blind study to admit that they did not adhere to the rules—that they took other medicine when the pain became too intense.

TOO LITTLE DATA, TOO LATE

Double-blind testing doesn't work with antibiotic therapy for essentially the same reason, but with exactly the opposite result: in cases of deeply entrenched rheumatoid arthritis, six months isn't long enough for the treatment to produce a beneficial effect—indeed, because of the Herxheimer reaction, during the test period the patient's condition can actually get worse.

That dual paradox is the essential flaw of the double-blind approach: the drugs that look good in the short term ultimately prove to be worse than worthless; the only medications that produce lasting benefits are the ones which six-month double-blind testing would be likely to eliminate at the start. In fact, one of the reasons for the failure of the so-called Boston Study of a few years ago, in which the effects of tetracycline therapy were analyzed in seventeen rheumatoid arthritics, was that it stopped too soon. (There were several other reasons: the low number of cases, the wrong frequency in administration of the antibiotic; and the fact that more than half the patients were receiving other medications at the same time.)

ALTERNATIVES

Recently a doctor in the Infectious Disease Institute of the National Institutes of Health isolated a strain of mycoplasma from the joint fluid of a human with rheumatoid arthritis. Such isolations are no longer unusual and several others, including ourselves, have done the same thing. What was unusual was that the NIH doctor then inoculated a chimpanzee with this human strain of mycoplasma and induced arthritis in the animal. This animal model provides the perfect opportunity to prove cause and effect and to provide a means for controlling drug testing.

It would be far better to return to the method we used in the past: evaluating a drug over a five-year period, and comparing this with data already accumulated on the effect of gold for the same period of time. Such a comparison has been made with data supplied from our Arthritis Institute. Ninety-nine patients who had been treated with the antibiotic approach over a five-year period were selected for this study. Most of these patients had previously discontinued standard remedies, because they became toxic or ineffective. The data were examined by an independent statistical group who agreed that our results were valid. A comparison was made with the published data on a hundred patients who were treated with gold for a period of five years. More than 80 percent of our patients who had been treated with antibiotics were still improving after five years, whereas only 10 percent of the patients treated with gold were still on the drug. The other 90 percent of the gold patients had dropped out for the familiar reason: the gold had either become toxic or had lost its effectiveness.

In the case of AIDS research, there has been bitter, protracted debate regarding the need or justification for double-blind controls, and such controls are now no longer required in evaluating therapeutic results. A method of testing arthritis drugs that proceeds in the same manner as testing for AIDS medications would compare the failures and successes of different compounds in the same patients, not just for six months but for five years. This empirical approach would produce test information that is more relevant, far safer, and much more reliable than the double-blind method. It would not only reveal drugs that work, but exclude drugs that provide false hope—which in the long run only worsens the disease by increasing the stress from uncertainty and failure.

THE PRICE

The search for new, nonsteroidal anti-inflammatory drugs without toxic side effects and with the same pain-relieving qualities as cortisone has been enormously expensive, and the cost of the research has to be included in the retail price of the drugs. Many of the new compounds used for the treatment of arthritis were found to be toxic after they gained approval through six-month double-blind tests—and some of these delayed reactions proved to be lethal. Gold has been found to cause kidney trouble, and the newest form, oral gold, has been shown to suppress the formation of platelets and cause uncontrollable bleeding. Plaquenil has caused retinal damage, and penicillamine, which seemed to be remarkably effective when first used, has caused suppression of bone marrow in some people—and some deaths. The immunosuppressive drugs, such as methotrexate, have been found to damage the liver and sometimes the lungs.

Such complications have required intense monitoring of these drugs by the rheumatologist, ophthalmologist, and other specialists, all at considerable expense to the patient. Add the price of the drugs themselves, frequent laboratory tests, and costly treatments of the complications when they do occur, and a new perspective emerges on arthritis: its total cost to America is becoming far greater than that of the whole Vietnam War.

Fortunately, the risks associated with the standard treatments for arthritis are beginning to gain recognition at last and the circle is coming around again to a basic approach to the disease process. Medicine is getting back to where it was in the early 1950s, before the cortisone revolution. We are now standing at a crucial intersection in the quest for safety and security for the arthritic. We must continue in the right direction, focusing on the infectious concept with vigor, determination, and open-mindedness, qualities notably lacking in the past thirty years. Of the several hundred grants that have been made for arthritis research, less than a dozen have funded programs to probe the infectious theory.

One factor which has played a major role in the reversal of this inequity has been the appearance of Lyme disease.

CHAPTER 21

Lyme Disease: A Portrait of Infectious Arthritis

The formula for any good story is that it must have a beginning, a middle, and a conclusion, and at present Lyme disease is the form of arthritis that comes closest to meeting that requirement; the model it provides for future researchers should eventually lead to a full library of happy endings. For most people, including lovers of detective stories and romantics who like to see everything properly disposed of and explained in the end, the story of Lyme disease is a classic thriller. For diehard advocates of the metabolic theory of rheumatoid arthritis, however, the final chapter brings some very unsettling news.

The first reported cases of Lyme disease were in 1975, in the town on the eastern shore of the Connecticut River that gives the affliction its name. Two mothers called the state health department to say that their children had just been diagnosed as having rheumatoid arthritis, and they suspected an epidemic. Juvenile rheumatoid arthritis can be a very serious disease, and when the department looked into the situation they found that indeed there were several other cases in the vicinity, as well an inordinate number of adult cases reported in the same period.

The health authorities called Yale University School of Medicine and spoke with a postdoctoral fellow in rheumatology named Allen Steere. Steere took on the puzzle. He started by calculating that the thirty-nine children and twelve adult cases diagnosed to that date represented a rate of incidence a hundred times higher than normal for the size of the population. Moreover, in areas where cases of the disease clustered—heavily wooded rural sites—the rate was ten thousand times higher than it should have been. Steere then identified several important features of the epidemic. From the pattern of dates on which families and neighbors showed their first symptoms, he concluded that it was a summertime affliction and that it was not highly contagious, which is to say that those afflicted were not catching it from one another but from some other source. A clue to that unknown source was found in the fact that a quarter of the victims recalled having an unusual rash a couple of days to a month before the first signs of arthritis, and the distribution and form of the rash suggested the bite of a crawling insect or spider.

PATTERN RECOGNITION

Steere also discovered that the same skin rash pattern had been reported in Europe in 1909, although without the subsequent arthritis, and that it had been traced to the bite of a tick, *Ixodes ricinus*. Some decades later, cases of that same rash pattern in Europe were treated with penicillin and cured, from which scientists inferred that the active agent in 1909 had been a bacterial infection. Accordingly, an attempt was made to isolate bacteria from the synovial fluid of several victims of the Lyme epidemic, but nothing showed up.

A couple of years after he started, Steere had a piece of extraordinary luck: one of the people who came down with the disease in 1977 not only recalled having been bitten by a tick—but he had saved it. Steere sent the tick up to Harvard, where it was identified as *Ixodes dammini*, a close cousin of the

European protagonist of seventy years earlier. Distribution studies subsequently established *Ixodes dammini* as the likely vector, or carrier, of Lyme disease.

SPIROCHETE INFECTION

That still didn't explain what Lyme disease was. Many ticks were gathered from the wild, but studies of their organs and digestive systems were no more productive than the earlier work with human joint fluid. Four years later, however, other scientists researching an outbreak of Rocky Mountain spotted fever opened the digestive system of an *Ixodes dammini* and found that it was filled with spirochete bacteria. They knew that the tick was the prime suspect in Lyme disease, and they guessed that the spirochete was the long-sought infectious agent. Subsequently the connection was proven. DNA studies showed the spirochete was a new species, which was named *Borrelia burgdorferi* after the researcher who first saw it.

Researchers who studied Lyme disease under a grant from the National Institutes of Health have identified three clinical stages, although not all patients demonstrate all stages. The first, showing up within a few days to a month after the bite, can include migratory rash, fatigue, fever, chills, and aches. The second stage can include irregular electrical activity in the heart muscle, showing up as shortness of breath, dizziness, and palpitations. The third stage is arthritis, sometimes accompanied by disorientation and memory loss. All three of those stages can vary widely, and Lyme disease is frequently misdiagnosed, often as Alzheimer's or multiple sclerosis.

KNOCKING IT OUT

Even if treatment waits until the third stage, either penicillin or tetracycline is still effective in knocking out most cases, although the NIH-sponsored researchers found that some

entrenched incidents require that the antibiotics be administered intravenously. They also noted that several physicians treating the arthritic stage of the disease had encountered the
Herxheimer effect, in which the symptoms became temporarily
worse once treatment began, and they suspected that this reaction was another important clue. Subsequent laboratory tests
showed that the Herxheimer effect probably results from the
release of powerful agents from the walls of the dying bacteria as
they are attacked by the antibiotic; these, in turn, stimulate the
host body's immune defense mechanism.

That same chain reaction accounts for the Herxheimer effect
in every other rheumatoid form of arthritis, whether the invading agent is a spirochete, streptococcus, or mycoplasma.

Of course, the chain reaction of rheumatoid arthritis doesn't
begin or end with the Herxheimer effect. In the more common
forms of arthritis, for example, we have known for a long time
that mycoplasmas localize, and that if you can get them out of
the joints, in most cases the condition will improve. We also
know, even accounting for the Herxheimer effect, that if we're
progressing at a good rate and the patient is getting better, it
very often happens that some other bacterial antigen will enter
the picture and make matters worse again. What has occurred
in those instances is that the antigens from the mycoplasma or
some other disease agent have sensitized the area in question,
so that future incidents now have an easy place to happen.

When the stage is set in that way, lots of other factors can get
into the act. Medication and foods can become serious problems,
for example, as the sensitized body begins to reject them. Sinus
troubles or kidney problems can appear. Antigens of many different types can enter the picture and create chaos.

SLEEPER

One of the sleeping antigens that is very hard to measure is
streptococcus. It has been well established that the toxins from
streptococci, as well as those from mycoplasmas, have an

affinity for joints. We have found in the course of taking comprehensive histories of our patients that a tremendous number of them have had severe troubles with their sinuses or their tonsils or their ears, or have had scarlet fever or rheumatic fever—all streptococcal conditions. Strep is an organism that is very susceptible to penicillin, which is why rheumatic fever and scarlet fever are no longer the terrible menaces they were a generation ago. But even after it has been knocked out as a source of infection, streptococcus hangs on for years—in tonsils, around teeth, and in other hiding places—not causing infection, but serving as another source of antigen, or toxin, with that demonstrated specificity for joints.

In treating rheumatoid arthritis, when a physician gets to the point with tetracycline therapy that the mycoplasmas have been substantially reduced and further progress appears to be limited, it makes sense to probe the possibility that streptococcus is complicating the process. If a titer of streptococcal antibodies indicates that their levels are elevated, then both the mycoplasma and the strep can be treated at the same time, continuing tetracycline for the former and using ampicillin for the latter.

Nothing about rheumatoid arthritis is simple, and it doesn't necessarily stop there; the streptococcus often alters its form (see discussion of L-form in Chapter 18), which further compounds the problem. Treatment of the strep then takes one kind of medication, and treatment of the altered form requires yet another.

THE INFECTIOUS ALLERGY

All of these scenarios follow the pattern of infectious allergies, which is one of the central processes of all forms of rheumatoid arthritis and which must be addressed in their treatment. Lyme disease is harder to cure the longer it remains untreated; when the allergic reaction has been given enough time to become securely established, the resistance to therapy can be multiplied many times over. The same applies to all other forms of rheumatoid arthritis.

Finally, for those who like a moral with their short stories, it should be acknowledged that Lyme disease proves once again that there is no such thing as a panacea in dealing with mankind's oldest disease. Tetracycline may be all a doctor could ask for in treating many other forms of rheumatoid arthritis—even most of them—but by itself it is still not the whole answer.

The whole answer is in the one area that has received the least attention in the past forty years and that has finally been illuminated by the brilliant research which solved the puzzle of Lyme disease: a complete understanding of the causes of rheumatoid arthritis and of the mechanism by which it occurs.

CHAPTER 22

Tomoka: The First Animal Model

T omoka is a silver-back gorilla, and he lives at the National Zoo in Washington, D.C. Twenty-six years ago, Tomoka made headlines as the second gorilla ever to be born in captivity in the United States, the fourth such captive birth in the world.

Despite the national attention he received by virtue of his origins, Tomoka is a perfect example of the fickleness of fame; by the time he was five years old, most of his adoring public had abandoned him and he was a has-been. His growth had stopped at a frail 150 pounds, and he sat in the corner of his cage rubbing his joints and looking miserable. A terribly sick gorilla in the zoo represents the same kind of liability as a waiting room full of sick, depressed humans in a doctor's office—it is a downer, and reflects poorly on those in charge. Nobody likes to spend his free time witnessing that kind of embarrassment. In addition, the animal was suffering from a great deal of pain and had not responded to more than twenty different remedies used for the treatment of arthritis in humans.

We were called by zoo officials and asked if we would be interested in having pathological material to study when they put him to sleep, which was planned to be carried out in a few days. We asked to see Tomoka, examine him, and do studies of his blood before they carried out their plans, and they agreed.

It soon became clear that we were seeing the first model of human rheumatoid arthritis ever encountered in an animal. Our success in treating humans with the antibiotic approach was well known in the Washington community, and with some persuasion the zoo officials allowed us to treat the gorilla with intravenous tetracycline; we in turn agreed that if there was no response, then they should carry out their plans. I did point out that it might take some time before Tomoka showed signs of improvement, and they agreed to accept this arrangement.

Tomoka was treated with intravenous tetracycline by drip every two weeks. Although he got worse at the outset of therapy, he gradually began to get better, gaining in strength and then in weight. We have now followed Tomoka for more than twenty years. His flare reactions progressively lessened in both frequency and intensity over approximately a three-year period, and he has remained completely well for the balance of that time. He is now a healthy, strong, very active, full-grown gorilla. He has only one toe that bears the remains of some cartilaginous destruction, and that in no way hinders his activity.

Since Tomoka's case was reported, we have been in touch with a great many zoos which have told us of similar cases. We have advised our treatment, and there are now more than thirty gorillas that we know of that are doing well under this program. We also know of two gorillas that were treated by standard methods and died; we are not sure of the cause of death.

Dr. Dan Laughlin, a veterinarian at the Chicago Zoo, told me of the zoo's success in treating one of their gorillas who had arthritis similar to Tomoka's. Dr. Laughlin came to see me because of his own arthritis and I learned that he had seen a great deal of arthritis in elephants, which was his area of special interest. Dr. Harold Clark, our research associate, has pursued laboratory studies of the elephants and a number of strains of mycoplasma comparable to those in the gorillas have been detected by mycoplasma complement fixing reactions in the blood.

Tomoka's care and the results of his treatment have attracted a lot of attention as well as controversy, although among veterinarians there is only enthusiasm. An article in the *Washington Post* in April 1984 says of these veterinarians, "They are ... convinced that Brown's treatment ... has essentially eliminated rheumatoid arthritis as a major threat to zoos and circuses."

CHAPTER 23

How Arthritis Happens: The Mechanism

The idea that there is a viruslike agent or some kind of invisible infectious component in the tissues affected by arthritis had its start in work done at the Rockefeller Institute between 1936 and 1939. The results of that work were published first in a brief article in *Science* in 1939, and then elaborated some ten years later in the rheumatic disease section of *Post Graduate Medicine and Surgery*. A paper by Dr. Louis Dienes and Howard Weinberger entitled "Experimental Arthritis: Pleuropneumonia-like Organisms and their Possible Relation to Articular Disease" spoke of the L-form of bacteria as "an invisible, filterable form that may exist after the parent germ disappears."

THE L-FORM

I had arrived at a similar understanding through my own observations in the late 1930s, but from a different point of view. I had gone to the Rockefeller Institute to try to disclose the presence of some virus or infection in rheumatic tissues, using embryonated hen's eggs as the tissue on which to grow the organisms. All of my results had been negative for the first three or four months; I had inoculated hundreds of eggs, and nothing at all had shown up on the membrane. Finally, when something did appear, it turned out to be the so-called L-form, or what we thought was bacteria. (The L-form took its name from the Lister Institute in London, where it was first described by Dr. Emmy Klieneberger. It was not until some years later that a committee of the American Microbiological Society decided to give this class of organisms a more formidable name. *Mycoplasma* derives from the Latin base words for fungus and fluid.)

By isolating a strain of the L-form organism from a Bartholin cyst, which occurs on female labia, Dienes became the first researcher to observe it in humans. I was the first one to find an L-form strain in joints and to connect it to arthritis.

WHY THINGS SOMETIMES GET WORSE BEFORE THEY GET BETTER

I was asked to write a discussion of the Dienes-Weinberger paper, and I reported that we had observed this organism in a number of clinical situations. Seventeen patients, representing a wide variety of rheumatic diseases including rheumatic arthritis, rheumatoid spondylitis, chorea, erythema nodosum, and rheumatic fever, were treated with Aureomycin, a tetracycline derivative, because it had an effect on these organisms. As an interesting corollary, we noted that gold salts produced approximately the same result. And we were also impressed that when we started treating these patients with a tetracycline product (the Aureomycin), they invariably got worse before they started getting better—a phenomenon in medicine known as the Jarisch-Herxheimer reaction.

This discussion was the first linking in the entire medical literature of the Jarisch-Herxheimer effect with a tetracycline derivative in a rheumatic problem. Presumably the effect was due to the dislodging and breaking up of the mycoplasma and the releasing of antigen to a sensitized field. The effect showed a number of important principles at work. It demonstrated that the disease was a hypersensitive reaction, not to the drug itself but to the toxins that a germ creates in response to the drug's presence. It showed that the germ must indeed be invisible, as Dienes and Weinberger had suggested, because no other germs of such standard types as streptococcus and staphylococcus were isolable. And it opened the way to a chemical attack on the whole area of arthritis and rheumatic diseases.

HARD TO DO, HARD TO DUPLICATE

After our original research results were published in *Science* in 1939, our observations quickly became news. The *New York Times* ran a full page on the subject, and there was a lot of excitement among the media. But after a very short time, the excitement died.

The problem was that no one else was able to duplicate our results. This was thoroughly predictable; after all, it had taken me three months before I had been able to achieve those results in the first place, and other researchers tried it once or twice and gave up. When I left the Rockefeller Institute in 1939 and went back to Johns Hopkins to become chief resident in medicine, the school gave me a laboratory and eventually a fellow to pursue the subject further. I remained convinced that the subject was worth more work, but I found myself in a fast-shrinking minority in my conviction.

These original observations gave us a basis for looking at the possibility that rheumatoid arthritis was due to a kind of infectious allergy, and that mycoplasmas, unlike other germs that worked by invading the host, operated instead by sitting still in one place and giving off, in a pulsating fashion, something to which the body reacted. Because those emissions were irregular, there were periods when the disease was thoroughly quiescent and the person with arthritis would feel reasonably healthy. Conversely, there were other times—often associated with periods when the patient worked too hard or was under great stress or suffered an injury—when the hidden organism released toxins and the disease would flare up.

BREAKING THE EGG

It was one thing to infer the presence of mycoplasmas by observing their effects, but it was often quite another to study them at first hand. To begin with, they proved to be both extremely fragile and very good at hiding, not only on the host cell but within it. And if the research effort did anything to damage the area in which these tiny organisms were located, the mycoplasmas would quickly break up. When that happened, it was similar to an egg breaking in the refrigerator, with the remnants running everywhere.

Over the years, we studied what happens when the mycoplasmic egg is broken. We learned, eventually, that the toxin leaving the organism is not, in itself, particularly vicious; if it were, we realized that it would make the patient terribly sick, since a little bit of the toxin is escaping from the mycoplasma all the time. Instead, we came to understand that when the toxin is released over a period of months or years, it creates a reception by "fixed tissue antibodies" that are ready to react to these toxins every time they appear.

The way in which the body becomes sensitized to mycoplasmas is similar to the way in which it learns to react to poison ivy. First-time visitors to the United States could take a shower in poison ivy resins, and the only thing most of them would get from it would be sticky. Until the body produces an antibody or allergen, there's no reaction. By the same token, one could expect that it would take prolonged exposure to mycoplasma toxins before the stage would be properly set for a reaction to occur. Many of us could be carrying mycoplasmas from childhood—from an old infection, perhaps from viral pneumonia—that are ticking away inside our bodies, just waiting for that process to play itself out.

We also learned early on that mycoplasmas have a unique affinity for certain parts of the body, and they attach themselves there like no other germ. Most of what we know in that respect comes from work performed by other scientists on animals such as swine, chickens, and turkeys, particularly the research conducted by Albert Sabin on laboratory mice in which mycoplasmas were isolated, injected into the animals' bloodstreams, and headed unfailingly to the joints.

MYCOPLASMAS AND JOINTS

The history of science is filled with stories of major discoveries which seem so obvious in retrospect that one marvels at how long they remained unknown. The development of penicillin in 1928, for example, was greeted with universal delight, followed almost immediately by chagrin among several generations of physicians who, like Alexander Fleming, had observed the effects of mold on cultures growing in a petri dish but unlike him had inferred nothing useful from what they saw.

It is a lot easier to recognize a cure than to understand the mechanism of a disease, especially when the disease is as complex as rheumatoid arthritis. That principle may help us to understand why some of the most elemental properties of arthritis went unrecognized for decades after they should have become perfectly obvious. And it may help as well in explaining why arthritis has such a sorry history of "cures," many of which have proven more destructive than the disease itself.

The affinity of mycoplasmas for the tissue and fluid of the joints is just one such uniform factor that no one seemed to have noticed before, despite ample opportunities going back at least to the 1890s. At that time, a devastating epidemic of arthritis and pneumonia, called pleuropneumonia bovis, swept through the cattle herds of Europe, causing incredible mortality and raging across to the eastern end of Siberia. It was caused by a germ called *Streptobacillis moniliformis*, which grows in great chains in the culture media—and produces L-forms that mimic mycoplasmas. Scientists cultured the larger germ and, at a hundred magnifications on a microscope stage, they observed colonies of what looked like dozens and even hundreds of tiny fried eggs, unquestionably satellites to the parent organism. While they recognized that the satellite derived from the host, much as the moon originated in the area of the earth now occupied by the Pacific Ocean, they failed to understand that the fried eggs were another form of the same lethal agent and were at least as potent as the long strands of ropelike streptobacilli.

The satellite concept is useful in another way in appreciating how the mechanism of arthritis has remained so elusive. Let's suppose that a visitor from Mars were to visit the moon and ask the moon where it came from. If the moon could point to the earth and say, "I came from there," the Martian visitor shouldn't have much difficulty with that answer. But now suppose that something cataclysmic had happened after the moon was formed, and the earth was no longer there. It becomes a lot harder for the visitor to say, "I see," when the thing that he might have seen has disappeared.

THE GREAT DEBATE

This phenomenon of a kind of metamorphosis or variation from the streptobacillus into the L-form or mycoplasma— coupled with the disappearance of the original form—led to a tremendous debate between Dienes in the United States and Klieneberger in London. Dienes said that the mycoplasma derived from the streptobacillus with which it was originally intermingled and was another phase of the same creature. Klieneberger said the two phases were separate organisms, much as a pony is separate from a horse. The argument took on the aspects of a theological debate, Klieneberger representing the redoubtable Lister Institute, where the L-form had first been identified and after which it was named, and Dienes, on the other side of the ocean, releasing his arrows from behind the mighty ramparts of Harvard University.

Unhappily, as this battle raged, I found myself somewhere near the metaphoric equivalent of Bermuda, right in the middle. In my work at Johns Hopkins, we had recently isolated some streptobacillus from the joint fluid of a man who had been bitten by a rat. Streptobacillus was known to be carried by rats, and I recognized that the outcome of the debate would have profound implications for my work, and possibly vice versa.

In due course, Jack Nunemaker joined me and we were able to demonstrate that the L-form was a variant of the original streptobacillus organism, and we had reason to believe that all bacteria could indeed go into separate invisible forms. We showed that a germ could enter a state in which it could become invisible, pass through a filter, and then return to the parent form. It was a whole new world of subclinical phenomena, a world in which things could appear and disappear, take new shapes, be at once different and the same—the biochemical equivalent of solid ice changing into water or steam and back again as circumstances require. Was it possible, from the long persistence of the forms in tissues, that bacterial allergy would evolve?

ENTER, THE SHADOW

This view changed the way we looked at certain kinds of disease. A person could have osteomyelitis, for example, and the staphylococcus that caused it could clear up, leaving the patient fully healed, with no sign of the infectious agent no matter how many times it was cultured. But if that person then were to be given a lot of cortisone—enough to interfere with his immune mechanism—all of a sudden the old staphylococcus would come back to life again with a vengeance, returning to the visible world from out of nowhere, from out of the persisting invisible L-form.

When one accepts that Lamont Cranston is also the Shadow and can move back and forth between at least two states and maybe among several, it is easy to see implications for our understanding the mechanism of other diseases than arthritis. Multiple sclerosis, for example, and amyotrophic lateral sclerosis (Lou Gehrig's disease) have all kinds of invisible but seemingly infectious states.

From that point on, we continued looking for the L-form, or mycoplasma, separate from any other organism. I realized that we couldn't do this by inoculating tissues of animals or tissue cultures, because that procedure would leave us open to the suspicion of contamination. So instead we worked with exudates from the body and the blood directly into culture media, without using animals, eliminating the risk that we would pick up anything along the way. For thirty years, we tried to grow mycoplasmas from joint fluid, knowing from the start that they are extremely fragile structures and very difficult to cultivate outside the body.

LEARNING ABOUT MYCOPLASMA

Mycoplasmas are not viruses. True viruses require living cells in which to grow. Mycoplasmas are somewhere between a virus and a bacterium, but the real difference is that they contain RNA and DNA and are self-contained, living units. That difference is important, but their similarities to some viral forms were to prove instructive as well, especially when we began looking for mycoplasmas inside the human body and within living cells. A couple of years ago, armed with new, state-of-the-art equipment for electron microscopy and protein fractionation, we set about doing just that.

We were also armed with a formidable new director of research. Millicent Coker-Vann, with a Ph.D. in biochemistry in viral immunology, came to the Arthritis Institute from the National Institutes of Health, where she had been working in particular with the slow virus group. Although she had been connected with the NIH for more than a decade, along the way she taught for two years at the University of Ife in Nigeria, spent seven months as a fellow at the Max Planck Institute in West Germany, and received a research grant from the Rockefeller Foundation.

Breaking down the proteins of the body is somewhat like unwrapping a cocoon. Under Dr. Coker-Vann's guidance, we soon found that by fractionating the protein, we could easily layer off the mycoplasma antigen fraction, draw it off, put it in a rabbit, and develop antibodies against it which would match those of the patient. In a very short time, we were able to complete the circle back to the patient without having to isolate any of the elements from animal intermediaries.

Now we had both the mycoplasma antigen and the antibody in relation to the disease. We have found higher concentrations of both the antigen and the antibody in the joint fluid than in the blood. And the levels of both antigen and antibody have been noted to decrease following intravenous antimycoplasma therapy.

Early in the course of pursuing the new fractionation technology, we found that it wasn't necessary to have the whole living mycoplasmic organism to provoke the reaction in a joint or tissue. Our studies proved what we had previously been able to assume only by inference—that just the fragments of mycoplasmas were sufficiently potent to create a powerful antigenic reaction, causing the host to produce antibodies in reaction to their presence.

THE EVIDENCE ACCUMULATES

Over the course of time, we accumulated a larger and larger body of evidence that mycoplasmas were indeed the mechanism for rheumatoid arthritis.

First of all, only antimycoplasma drugs had any impact on

rheumatoid disease, except in those instances where there was a strong streptococcal connection. Ampicillin may be needed to lower the streptococcal antigen level and reduce symptoms. Tetracyclines were the only group of antibiotics we could find that suppress mycoplasma growth in the laboratory, and they were the only ones that seemed to improve the arthritis patients' conditions—unless there were other bacterial complications which added to the sensitizing process.

A further body of data was derived from studies of the other medicines, potions, and old wives' cures that have been used over the years to combat arthritis. Quinine is a long-time remedy for arthritis and a ubiquitous component of patent medicines that goes back centuries; it was used by our great-grandparents for backaches and rheumatism—so much so that many of our ancestors developed serious quinine allergies. We demonstrated, not surprisingly, that quinine has a specific effect on mycoplasmas, as does Plaquenil (hydroxychloroquine sulfate), another antimalarial substance to which quinine is closely related. Gold has also been found effective in suppressing mycoplasma growth, explaining its effectiveness in arthritis. We demonstrated the antimycoplasmic action of gold nearly forty years ago. Copper salts were first used by J. Forestier at about the same time he discovered the value of gold in rheumatoid disease, and he particularly noted their beneficial effect on rheumatoid arthritis; again, we demonstrated the ability of this substance to suppress mycoplasma growth. By the same token, it has been observed that copper bracelets react with perspiration to form copper salts, and work in Australia recently proved that those copper salts can penetrate the skin, which would explain the popularity of this preventive talisman from as long ago as the time of the ancient Romans.

Collectively, our observations confirmed a pattern in which mycoplasma could be seen as the consistent offender in the process by which rheumatoid arthritis occurs, and that pattern more than justified our efforts to isolate it.

We are also trying to "tag" the mycoplasma organism so we can see where it combines with human tissue. Tagging is a procedure by which the element under study is labeled with a tracer which signals its presence in microscopy. The reason for this approach is that without tagging, once the mycoplasma enters tissue, it is lost to view and can't be identified with any certainty, even with the electron microscope.

POINTING TO THE CAUSE OF RHEUMATOID ARTHRITIS

Regardless of what we learn about the final pieces of the rheumatoid arthritis puzzle in the time just ahead, I believe we already know enough about the mechanism—inferentially and from direct observation in our laboratory research, and from forty years of clinical experience—to state with certainty that mycoplasmas are the primary infectious agent, and that tetracycline therapy is the only effective therapy to reach toward the cure of rheumatoid arthritis.

The cause of rheumatoid arthritis is an antigenic substance which operates not as an invader, in the way of germs, but as the trigger for an internal allergic response, releasing toxins intermittently to a sensitized area, subsiding then reappearing We know that antibodies are transported throughout the body by white blood cells and platelets, much as smoke jumpers are carried by an airplane from one brush fire to the next. It is by this means that arthritis migrates, in the knee one day and in the shoulder or the back the next: the antigen builds up in the shoulder, and the antibody that was busy counteracting it in the knee moves on to the new battlefield, leaving the knee to a brief season of peace.

DEFLATING SOME MYTHS

Consider the alternatives. If one is to believe that rheumatoid arthritis is just a hereditary problem, or that it is due to stress or nutritional deficits or aging or a deficiency in the body's natural supply of cortisone, how is it possible to explain, for example, that the condition flares up the day before a storm comes?

One way in which myths are preserved is by the denial of evidence that would disprove them. Advocates of the genetic, nutritional, stress, aging, and cortisone-deficiency schools of arthritis simply dismiss the indications that arthritis is barometrically poised by calling them old wives' tales. But Dr. Joseph Hollander, the head rheumatologist at the University of Pennsylvania in Philadelphia, did a study some years ago of the effects on rheumatoid disease of barometric pressure, along with such other factors as temperature, humidity, and oxygen. He got volunteers to stay in sealed, climatically controlled rooms, writing their impressions of how they felt from hour to hour as he worked various subtle changes in their environment. It can be assumed that some of the changes, such as in humidity, might have been detectable through normal sensory means, but most of the changes were not. Hollander concluded, on the basis of excellent clinical evidence, that environment does indeed make a measurable difference in one's sensitivity to rheumatic disorders. Two factors were found to cause flare-ups: a sudden drop in barometric pressure, and the presence of high humidity in conjunction with such a drop. Both of them are common atmospheric characteristics prior to a storm. The barometric effect fits our concept perfectly by promoting a sudden release of antigen to a sensitized area.

I have always asked new patients about their experience with changes in weather, and also about their sensitivity to changes in the seasons. It has been well known for many years that patients with rheumatoid arthritis experience a higher incidence of flare-ups in the late spring and early fall. Very little work has been done in understanding the impact of seasonal changes on disease, although the increased incidence of depression that comes with the arrival of fall has been widely noted for a number of years, perhaps because it is supported by a measurable indicator in the form of a corresponding rise in the suicide rate. Our clinical experience with rheumatoid arthritis has shown that it, too, is subject to seasonality.

One other old wives' tale is worth examining for the clues it might provide to the arthritis mechanism, and that is the ancient belief that the pain in arthritic joints can be relieved by bee venom. This rather painful therapy is commonly practiced by the residents of New Hampshire, as indeed it is by rural folk throughout the world. New Hampshire happens to be favored by its proximity to Boston, and many members of the immense medical community in that city spend their weekends among the rustics in the Granite State, observing their ways.

As might be expected, visiting doctors who hear about bee-sting therapy warn its practitioners that they are risking a fatal reaction to the venom—which is indeed the case—and they usually dismiss the claims for its efficacy out of hand. But the claims persist. Following a hunch, several years ago Dr. Harold Clark in our laboratory sent away for some bee venom and our microbiologist, Jack Bailey, tested it against various strains of mycoplasma. It proved to be a very potent suppressor of their growth.

I am happy to report that the bee venom story isn't likely to end there. Some researchers in Great Britain have been studying its effects on arthritis and attempting to dissect it chemically, aiming toward the possibility that they will be able to separate the curative component from the part that creates the sting. It would be my own guess that the cure and the sting are one and the same thing, but I am delighted to see more research that is directed toward the mechanism by which arthritis occurs.

In the main, the history of arthritis research over the past four decades has been one of frustration, suffering, or serial disappointment as one miracle cure after another failed to live up to its early promise. The reason for those failures always comes down to one basic flaw: no major disease has ever been cured before science has first developed an understanding of how it works.

COMPLETING THE PUZZLE

At long last, the main parts of the puzzle are falling into place, and our understanding of the fundamental mechanism of rheumatoid arthritis is now nearly complete. There are still many aspects that need to be explored, but this new framework allows us to approach them in a different light, no longer dismissing the disease as hopeless and without a known cause. This is the framework within which arthritis occurs. The process taking place within that framework is often far more complicated than I have shown, and some of its parts are still only dimly seen. There may well be other bacteria that contribute to the process of arthritis once it starts. Many people with tonsillitis or bad teeth or kidney infections may experience flares in their arthritis from these additional sources of antigen, just as people with noses that are sensitized to ragweed will find that they have also become sensitive to such other stimuli as house dust and feathers. But as surely as the primary cause of hay fever is ragweed, the starting point for arthritis is mycoplasmas.

Once a person's joints have become sensitized to mycoplasmas, which move in and settle there, other antigens can move into the same neighborhood and compound the problem. If there is a strong history of streptococcal infection (rheumatic fever, scarlet fever, frequent strep throats with ear and sinus complications) or a strongly positive ASO (streptococcal antibody level), additional treatment with appropriate antistreptococcal medication as a therapeutic probe is often indicated. Regardless of these other factors, however, the basis for the initial sensitivity is still mycoplasma, and if the mycoplasma can be removed, the sensitivity level of the rest of the body can be lowered as well and the other factors become more manageable. This framework provides the conceptual core for at last proving the cause of rheumatoid arthritis and finding its cure.

CHAPTER 24

How Do People Get Rheumatoid Arthritis?

R heumatoid arthritis is an acquired disease, but the way people get it—and whether they get it—is determined by factors that are as complex as arthritis itself.

The principal complication is in the fact that rheumatoid arthritis involves a bacterial allergy. One of the characteristics of bacterial allergies is that the allergic process is so powerful, the body isolates the germ and keeps it from being transmitted to others.

A good model for that phenomenon is undulant fever, or brucellosis, a disease acquired from cattle or swine. Undulant fever is highly contagious among such livestock, and if one animal catches it, the disease spreads through the herd like wildfire. Man can contract undulant fever by drinking milk from an infected animal, but it has never been known in the history of medicine that the disease has been transmitted from one human to another. I believe the reason is that man, unlike cattle and swine, is so reactive to the antigens made by brucellae that the reactive state walls it off and keeps it highly localized, not allowing it to become a contagious entity. The same thing happens with mycoplasmas.

TWO KINDS OF IMMUNITY

There are two main types of immunity: bloodstream immunity, in which certain factors in the blood protect us against particular diseases, and cellular immunity, in which the same protection is provided by the tissues of the body. The lack of cellular immunity is the reason children contract measles, whooping cough, chicken pox, mumps, and other so-called childhood disorders.

We know that mycoplasmas can be recovered from the genital tracts of women as a matter of routine. We look upon these organisms as parasites at that stage, but their presence at the end of the birth canal creates the possibility of a scenario in which the child can become infected and the relatively passive parasitic mycoplasma can eventually be transformed into an active agent of disease. If it happens that the mycoplasma enters the infant's body, the parasite could escape into the bloodstream and be carried to the joints, where it would attach to the synovial cells. It could remain in the parasitic stage indefinitely, ticking away, awaiting its time to turn into something far more serious.

RAISING SENSITIVITY

As the years go by, it is possible that these and other factors raise the body's level of sensitivity until it finally reaches a point where, on a localized basis, the stage is set for an allergic reaction. The allergy would be the result of the body responding to the persistent presence of these organisms by raising a defense to surround them. How the reaction is triggered is the subject of speculation: it might be an accidental bump or contusion, or severe mental stress—or in some cases it might be the trauma of childbirth. I have treated a great many patients who never suspected they had any kind of arthritis until they had gone through some such seemingly unrelated shock or stress. Almost invariably they have associated their disease with the event that acted as the trigger.

LIKE A VIRUS

If this linkage is correct, as I suspect it is, then the myco-plasma acts in the same way as a slow virus. Once the liberating event has set it off, it begins to create a reaction that walls it off even further to defend itself against attack by the body's immune system. That would explain why as arthritis becomes more entrenched it also becomes more severe.

This scenario also supports the thesis that all the rheumatoid forms of arthritis derive from essentially the same causes, as I believe they do, and that the many variations in the disease are simply a result of differing levels of allergy and reactivity in the hosts. Similarly, people who suffer from asthmatic allergies may react to dust in one case and feathers and pollens in another, but the allergy itself, regardless of the source, is the cause of their distress.

SOME DISTINCTIONS

The analogy with asthmatic allergies only holds up to a point, however; rheumatoid arthritis involves a living source of antigen which cannot be isolated from the patient in the way of ragweed or feathers. Bacterial antigens appear to have a physiological effect on things inside the body such as joints, muscles, nerves, the intestinal tract, and internal organs. The internal allergy is generally referred to as hypersensitivity to distinguish it from external allergies. Ordinary allergies affect the skin, the lungs, the eyes, and generally the outside of the body. Both can affect an intermediate ground, the gastrointestinal tract. External allergies come and go with changes in the environment, such as the seasons, or simply with cleaning the house or filtering the air. But internal hypersensitivities are built in and they persist, and the antigen from a bacterial source keeps coming, constantly or intermittently, and serves as a booster.

The reason housecleaning doesn't work with internal allergies is that they are so inaccessible, and as these hypersensitivity conditions get worse they get even harder to reach because the walls around them rise progressively higher. When viewed under the microscope, the areas of inflammation in the affected tissues are seen to be spotty, as though the body had erected a series of tiny fortresses around the causative factor.

At the very center of those fortresses are the mycoplasmas. Although their presence can be verified by other means such as protein fractionation, they usually can't be seen with certainty even by an electron microscope; the particles are so tiny that they are indistinguishable from the parts of the cell to which they attach. Even when a tissue is deliberately inoculated with mycoplasmas and the physician examines electron-microscopic sections of the infected cells, it is difficult to determine which of the particles are derived from mycoplasmas and which represent normal cellular constituents. Little wonder that the mycoplasmas' relationship to rheumatoid arthritis has eluded understanding for so long.

This near-invisibility is one more respect in which mycoplasmas are different from any other kind of disease agent. Even viruses, which are equally small, have what are called nuclear inclusions; the inclusion body in the nucleus of the cell for certain viruses is very distinctive, lining up in a crystalloid pattern of specks, and this "fingerprint" of one virus will be recognizably different from the pattern of another. Mycoplasmas don't line up in the nucleus.

LUPUS AND OTHER RHEUMATIC DISEASES

It is my belief that all of the rheumatic disorders, from the mildest arthritis to the most fatal form of lupus, involve mycoplasmas as a causative agent. There are two possible reasons for the same cause to produce such widely differing results: there are variations in how strongly the different tissues react against the organism, and there are some forms of mycoplasma that are more virulent than others.

There are other reasons for the immense number of variables in the arthritis family tree. Once the focus of sensitivity is established by the unique ability of the mycoplasma to attach to joints, other bacterial antigens can enter the picture and compound the problem. This is particularly true of the streptococcal antigen, which has a special affinity for sensitizing joints, as in rheumatic fever. Infected teeth, tonsils, sinuses, gallbladders, kidneys, and diverticula can contribute and often must be treated separately.

PNEUMONIA AS TRIGGER

The most vicious strain of mycoplasma that has been isolated to date and one whose antibody is very commonly present in the blood of rheumatoid arthritics is *Mycoplasma pneumoniae*, which causes viral pneumonia. I don't have any statistics on its incidence, but a lot of my patients over the years—far above the norm for the population as a whole—have suffered from walking pneumonia, an event which may well have supplied the trigger for a sudden upsurge in their arthritis.

THE L-FORMS

Another dimension of the question about the causes of arthritis that deserves far more laboratory research is all the other L-forms of bacteria. The L-forms so closely resemble mycoplasmas in the laboratory that at one time all mycoplasmas were referred to as L-form bacteria. If a researcher grows streptococci on a laboratory medium, adds penicillin to the medium, and kills the strep or other bacteria, he may see tiny, microscopic colonies of what look like clusters of fried eggs emerging from the remains of the germ, in exactly the same manner as mycoplasmas produce such colonies.

Microbiologists claim these particular fried eggs are not identical to mycoplasmas, and indeed there are some chemical differences. But they are the same in form and structure, and are specifically suppressed by tetracycline derivatives, as are mycoplasmas. They behave the same way, growing on the surface of media. Protein fractionation, electrophoresis, and other study techniques are just now starting to provide valuable clues to their exact nature and relationship to the arthritic process.

The payoff on such research could be enormous. In rheumatic fever, for example, streptococcus splits off L-forms which very likely get into connective tissue in joints, the heart muscle, and even heart valves. One cannot grow the strep from the joints or heart muscle or valves, but it is possible the L-form is in these places, setting up a local sensitivity without the strep itself being present. If so, that would explain the chronic, destructive changes that go along with rheumatic fever. It is curious that the damage to the joints is not permanent, but clears up when the disease comes to an end. But the damage to the kidney or heart that has been caused by this unknown factor—a strep antigen or whatever—does not clear up, and it can shorten life.

I wouldn't be at all surprised if research were to prove that when the L-form becomes fixed as a new entity, it becomes a mycoplasma. Phylogenetically, this could mean that back at the beginning of life, millions of years ago, there were only bacteria, and some of them evolved into the L-forms which later became mycoplasma, and some of them went in another direction to become parasites, amoebas, and other such organisms, adapting to changes in the environment.

ALL CONNECTIVE TISSUE DISEASES CAN BE TREATED EQUALLY

All diseases of the connective tissue are related to the same process that controls the rheumatoid forms of arthritis, and all respond, in greater or lesser degrees, to the same antibiotic approach to treatment. Lupus, which is a disease whose mortality figures are extremely unreliable because of a lack of continuity in observation, may kill as many as 75 percent of those who contract it. I have had consistently positive results in treating even very advanced cases with tetracycline, including several patients who have now reached what appears to be permanent remission.

One connective-tissue disease that proves the case for tetracycline even more incontrovertibly is scleroderma. It is a chronic hardening and shrinking of the connective tissues in which the skin turns to leather and, because the blood vessels are involved as well, the extremities become numb and cold. It affects the ectodermal portion of the esophagus so that eventually the patient loses the peristaltic motion that permits swallowing, and it can even invade the lungs and intestinal tract. It is a slow, progressive, inevitable death.

During the past few years, I have been sent a number of scleroderma patients from Athens, Alabama. They have all tested high for mycoplasma antibody levels—just as patients with lupus or rheumatoid arthritis or mixed osteo-rheumatoid arthritis or dermatomyositis do—and I have treated every one of them with tetracycline, just as I treat everyone who is suffering from these or any other disease of the connective tissues. And the scleroderma patients have all improved, some dramatically.

In the case of scleroderma, any improvement at all is dramatic, but these improvements are truly remarkable. The patients have increased their ability to swallow. The skin on their face and hands has started to loosen up and become supple again. Those who have been caught early don't have any further progression of the disease, and those who started late have begun to reverse their condition. The most striking result has been the reversal of widespread sclerodermatous pulmonary lesions.

A lot of doctors like to explain away any progress in rheumatoid arthritis or lupus by calling it natural remission. But they can't explain what happens with scleroderma as a natural remission because with that disease there isn't any such thing: under any other form of treatment the disease only goes one way, downward, and it doesn't stop until the patient is dead.

PINNING DOWN THE MYCOPLASMA

All these different types of connective-tissue disorders involve a circulating antibody against mycoplasma, but that is not to say that every patient proves positive for those antibodies every time he or she is tested. In those cases where the results are negative, as a rule all that is required to get a positive result is to follow the patient for a period until the antibody pops up again. The process of antibody circulation in rheumatoid arthritis or other such diseases is very similar to that in undulant fever, which is often very difficult to diagnose because of the wavelike periodicity of the antibody. The cyclical appearance and disappearance of a disease antibody is a widely recognized phenomenon of immunology. The Herxheimer effect, which is a toxic surge that follows the onset of treatment for mycoplasmic disorders, brings out the antibody in patients who have tested negative prior to treatment; as the treatment progresses, the antibody eventually tests negative again.

Eventually there will be a test for the antigen of mycoplasmas as well as for the antibody; diagnosticians will be able to look for the disease factor that creates the condition, rather than seeking an indication of the body's response. This is an area of research in which the Arthritis Institute is vigorously active. We have also noted a greater concentration of both antigen and antibody in joint fluid compared to the blood serum from the same patient.

In order to identify the antigen, it is first necessary to break down tissue, joint fluid, or blood into its serial protein fractions. Blood has any number of different proteins in it, one of which turns out to derive from mycoplasma. We have been measuring the direct signs of mycoplasma in the blood— either its toxins, particles of the germ, or the entire disease organism—to see whether it goes away when the patient is treated intravenously with tetracycline. And we have shown that it does.

We have also been collecting and analyzing data to look for a correlation between the dropoff of the antigen and the status of the symptoms as the patient is treated. Preliminary data are not sufficient to prove anything significant, but there is enough positive evidence to encourage further effort. One of the benefits of such a correlation, if it is proven, will be to provide an alternative to double-blind testing.

Not all of the information that has developed from fifty years of research and practice with connective-tissue disorders is of a kind that lends itself to statistical summary. In fact, I often feel that the source that has weighed most heavily over the long term, in helping me to understand what is involved in these diseases and in recognizing their patterns, is the kind of data that scientists characterize as anecdotal. In time, as it repeats itself over and over again, anecdotal data becomes progressively more substantive and meaningful. Perhaps more than any other aspect of learning, it has provided the deepest insights into the process by which arthritis happens to people.

That is the principal reason for the approach we have taken in the writing of this book.

CHAPTER 25

Scleroderma: Two Stories

DOYLE BANTA
Preacher/Educator/Businessman
Athens, Alabama

One morning about seven years ago, I noticed something strange on the inside of my left leg, just below the big muscle. It was about the size of a dime and it looked like a scar. I couldn't remember ever having injured my leg there, and I studied it, trying to figure out what it was.

Some time later I was in Birmingham to see my doctor about a thyroid problem, and I thought to show it to him. He couldn't figure it out either, but he said he wasn't a dermatologist; he suggested I put a little Vaseline on it and watch it.

A few months later it was about the size of a quarter and still growing, and it had started to change color, to get darker. I went over to a dermatologist in Decatur, and he diagnosed me as soon as he saw it. I can say that I'm one of the few cases that ever got a diagnosis so soon; I've met a lot of people since then who have scleroderma, lupus, multiple sclerosis, rheumatoid arthritis, and other things like that, and every one of them got diagnosed with something else before their doctors finally got it right.

The doctor told me a couple of interesting things about scleroderma: he said it's a rare disease, that it's even rarer for someone my age to get it, and rarer yet because I am a man. Most victims are twenty to forty years old, and 80 percent of them are women. He said to me, "I'll bet you thought you had cancer."

I said, "Well, I've seen enough cancer patients in my life, and I did think that's what it was."

"No, it's scleroderma," he said. "I'm not going to biopsy it because the wound will never heal up. But that's what it is."

I asked him what we should do about it, and he told me we couldn't do anything. He said he didn't know of anyone who had ever gotten over it, and he didn't know any place I could go to see a doctor who could give me any help. "But I will tell you this," he said. "Before it's over, you're going to wish it had been cancer instead."

I asked him why he said that. I told him the little amount I had on my leg didn't hurt at all, and I had heard that cancer was really painful.

"This will hurt you just as much as cancer. But the thing about cancer is that in a relatively short time it will wipe you out. Scleroderma won't; if a person is in good enough shape to begin with, it can last for as long as ten years."

"You think I'm going to live ten years with this disease before it kills me?" I asked.

"Not at your age," he answered. "I think you're probably going to live another three to five. And I wish you luck. If you find anybody that can do anything to help you, I'd sure like you to let me know."

We didn't make any plan that I would go back to him, because there didn't seem to be any point in it.

I've been preaching for forty-eight years, I've been on the board of Florida College in Tampa for twenty-four years, I've taught here in Athens, I know a lot of people through my insurance business, and I've traveled all over the country—so I get to meet a lot of people. I started hearing about folks who knew other people who had the same disease I had, and I talked with a lot of them, trying to find out what they were doing about it. We compared notes on how they first heard about it, and what their symptoms were. We kept in touch, and as the disease got further along for each of us, we'd tell each other our symptoms.

Over the next three and a half years, my scleroderma got really bad. By the middle of 1984 I didn't have any feeling in either leg from the middle of my thighs down to the ends of my toes. The skin on both legs was as dark as shoe leather, and just as hard, from about six inches above my knees all the way down. The pain was getting worse and worse; at night, it got so severe I would jump out of bed and walk for a long time to try to get some activity in the legs and both feet. I came on the idea that maybe heat would help, and so I started sleeping with two or three pairs of socks and a heating pad, and that provided some relief, but things were still very bad. With scleroderma, the blood vessels get squeezed from the thickening of the skin and the circulation gets cut off. I was afraid they were going to have to amputate my legs.

Another thing happened to me at about the same time: I began to get rheumatoid arthritis. After a while it got so painful, especially in the joints of my hands, that it sometimes hurt more than the scleroderma did. My doctor started me on steroids.

I prayed a lot. I decided I'd like to live longer, since I had a wife and two children and a daughter-in-law and six little grandkids. One Saturday I went to Huntsville, which I seldom do, to visit a friend who was planning on doing some building there. And while I was standing in his store, in walked a boy that I went to college with in Abilene, Texas, in 1941, someone I hardly ever see. We started talking, and he asked if I knew that a good friend of ours from years ago was suffering from cancer. "Nope, I hadn't heard that, and I'm mighty sorry," I said.

We talked about our friend for a while, and then I said, "Well, I've got something that's supposed to be even worse, and that's scleroderma."

"Man," he said, "I have good news for you."

"What's that?" I asked.

"There's a lady here in town, a good friend of ours, who has the same thing. She went to see a doctor somewhere in the northeast, and now she's in remission."

The lady's name was Cathryn Loftis. He gave me her telephone number and I called her. She listened to my story and told me just what to do. I then called my doctor, my doctor called Dr. Brown, and Dr. Brown said he was booked up for a whole year. But my doctor said I was a good friend of his and I was awful sick, and Dr. Brown changed things around to make room for me; three weeks later I was sitting in his office at the National Hospital in Arlington, Virginia. It was May of 1984.

There have been lots of changes in my scleroderma since Dr. Brown began his treatment. The dark leather has retreated halfway down my legs to several inches below my knees and keeps on getting smaller. There is still a dark area on one leg about the size of my hand, but otherwise the dark spots have gotten lighter and in some areas have gone away. The real difference is that I'm still alive, and both my doctor in Alabama and I agree that I wouldn't be if I hadn't heard about Dr. Brown. I live a hectic schedule in connection with my preaching, my insurance business, and the school, and I'm able to keep up with all of it. I still have a way to go, but I believe I'm headed for remission.

I stayed in the hospital in Virginia for twelve days that first visit, and Dr. Brown treated my scleroderma intravenously. He had me come back again in the late fall for another twelve days, and for two twelve-day visits the following year. In 1986 I had an unrelated problem with a kidney blockage that kept me in Alabama that May, but it cleared up and I went back to Dr. Brown for another stay that December.

Between visits to the hospital, I continue the treatment at home. I have done tremendously well, and everybody who knows me is just amazed at how I've recovered.

Fortunately, I have a lot of friends, and one of the great joys

I have gotten out of this is that I've sent forty people to Dr. Brown in the past three years, not just the people I met who have scleroderma, but also people with lupus and with rheumatoid arthritis, and every one of them has come back home and done what he said and is getting better. I stay in touch with them by telephone, and I know they all are just as amazed as I was at how Dr. Brown is able to get them better when everyone else had pretty much given up on them.

It also still amazes me that everyone I talk with who has scleroderma tells me the same thing about the way their previous doctors treated them: they just diagnosed the disease, got them started on steroids, and sent them home to die. Everyone I have ever sent to Dr. Brown is still alive. Not one of the lupus or scleroderma patients has died, and it doesn't look like anyone is going to, at least not from those diseases.

I'll be sixty-eight years old in January. Today I look ten years younger than I did three years ago. My skin looks healthy. Three years ago I was just dragging around, and today I'm on the go more than ever. In addition to the scleroderma getting so much better, there isn't a single trace of rheumatoid arthritis left in my hands or anywhere else, and my joints look as good as they ever have in my life. Dr. Brown told me that scleroderma and rheumatoid arthritis are both caused by a germ called a mycoplasma, and the same treatment with tetracycline helps get rid of them both. He sure was right. It's unbelievable to me how many people I've met who were at the brink of death, and he's brought them back to a good life.

CATHRYN LOFTIS
Housewife, Huntsville, Alabama

In 1976, I developed hepatitis and my recovery was very slow. My doctor followed me closely, and he said he thought the reason the hepatitis was giving me so much trouble was that there was something else there as well, something that he hadn't identified. He ordered a liver biopsy, and the lab kept it for two weeks; they couldn't figure out what it was either. The biggest symptom was my extreme fatigue. Most of the time I felt as though I had just run a marathon; if I got up at seven, by ten o'clock I'd have to go back to bed. It was a tremendous change from the way I used to be: I had played tennis a lot and was extremely active, and now I felt as though my head was in a vise and I walked around in a stupor. The doctor kept bringing me back for more tests and finally, after about a year and a half, he called me in one day and told me he thought I had a disease of the connective tissue.

I knew that wasn't good. A close friend of mine had a connective-tissue disease, one that affected all her muscles. The doctors had told her she had about seven years, and that was just about how long she lived.

One of the things the doctor noticed at that visit was that the skin on the ends of my fingers had gotten slick and unhealthy-looking. He asked me if I had noticed any changes in them over the past few months, and I had to admit I hadn't—I had been so distracted by my fatigue, I hadn't paid much attention to anything else. But my husband said that he saw the change, that the skin around the base of my fingernails seemed to be bowing out and that it had lost its natural color.

Our doctor sent me to a rheumatologist in Birmingham who examined me and said he thought I had an early case of scleroderma. By then the skin on my wrists was starting to thicken and I was seeing similar changes on either side of my face. That doctor sent me back to a dermatologist in Huntsville for a biopsy of one of the affected areas on my wrist. He told me to bring a picture of myself taken a year or more earlier, so there would be some basis for comparison in keeping track of the changes.

The dermatologist didn't want to do a biopsy when he first saw me, because he said he didn't think I had scleroderma. But after he looked more carefully at my face and hands he agreed there was some thickening so he went ahead. When he got back the lab report he told me he was sorry, that the test had been positive, and he sent me back to the rheumatologist. When I heard that, I knew it was serious, and so I was prepared for the worst. But I got a very different story at my next visit to the rheumatologist. He told me he was going to start me on Naprosyn (a nonsteroidal anti-inflammatory), and that he was sure I was going to handle the disease beautifully. He said there was no sign that the scleroderma had gotten inside my body yet, and the treatment was starting early enough that it probably never would touch any of my internal organs.

My local doctor had asked me to call him when I got back, and when he heard what the rheumatologist had told me he said, "But that just isn't so! It *will* affect your major organs and it will get progressively worse." I trusted and respected him, and knew he was telling me the truth.

Just a short time later, my husband, Lewis, was reading the paper and he saw a story about a Dr. Thomas McPherson Brown who had been invited to lecture at the University of Alabama in Huntsville. The story said that Dr. Brown had had remarkable success in treating rheumatoid arthritis, and Lewis wondered if he might have some ideas about scleroderma, which was in the same family. The next day I called our family doctor, and his response surprised me. "Of course he would! Of course you should talk to him! I read all about Dr. Brown's lecture, and I don't know why I didn't put two and two together. There's no question he's on to something with arthritis, and he's just the person you should be talking to about scleroderma." He was very distressed with himself for not thinking of it first and calling us.

He offered to telephone the Arthritis Institute in Washington for us, and he called back a short time later to say that Dr. Brown did indeed treat scleroderma, that he had had a lot of success with it, and that my doctor had already told his nurse to send my records to the National Hospital. We made an appointment for me to be in Washington three months later.

Meanwhile, we began to hear some extraordinary things

about Dr. Brown from other people around Huntsville. Lewis came home one evening and told me that a secretary at the Arsenal who had had rheumatoid arthritis so badly she couldn't type anymore had been treated by Dr. Brown, and her disease had nearly disappeared. I later heard that the wife of one of our county commissioners had been so sick with rheumatoid arthritis that she was in bed and her husband even had to feed her. She had been taken to see Dr. Brown, and some months later a friend had called her. The phone rang a long time, and just as the friend was about to hang up the woman answered. She sounded wonderful, and when the friend apologized for bothering her, she said it was no bother at all—she had just walked into the house from a trip to do her Christmas shopping. In every case, we were told that the improvement didn't take place overnight, that it took a lot of patience, but that Dr. Brown got nearly incredible results.

By the time I kept my appointment in Washington, in June of 1978, the evidence of the scleroderma on both my face and hands had become much more pronounced. The affected areas were alternately sickly white or flushed an unhealthy pink; I could see what the doctor called "the butterfly" of the disease on my face. My cheekbones looked gaunt and the skin over them was stretched unnaturally tight. I couldn't tolerate temperature variations in either direction by more than a few degrees. The first two fingers of my right hand had turned virtually to stone; I could have stuck a knife into either of them and I wouldn't have felt a thing. My energy level was so low that all I could do in a day was get out of bed in the morning and put on my clothes, and housework was out of the question. When we finally met Dr. Brown that night after I had checked into the hospital, Lewis asked him, "What does my wife have to look forward to?"

Dr. Brown smiled reassuringly and said, "Everything."

He told us we had to be patient, that the treatment didn't work overnight—that it could even take years—but that we could expect me eventually to be able to lead a perfectly normal life.

Three days after I started the antibiotic therapy I was taking a shower at the hospital and the rings on my left hand suddenly slipped off the finger. I told Dr. Brown about it right away; I couldn't believe the tetracycline had already had such a powerful effect on the swelling of the scleroderma. He was pleased, but he told me the swelling would return and that I shouldn't be disappointed when that happened. He warned me that it would take a total of three years before I saw any really significant difference, and for the first six months of his treatment I was going to feel worse and I would test worse.

I'm not sure how much worse I really felt in the next six months, but there's no doubt he was right that I didn't get any better during that time. I was still terribly fatigued, and I had almost no energy for anything except getting up and going back to bed. When the six months were up I went back to Washington for more treatments and another set of tests, and sure enough the scores were worse than when I had entered the hospital for my first stay the previous June. But on the visit after that, also as Dr. Brown had predicted, the results began to improve. And it kept on like that. Two years and seven months after he had first treated me, I noticed a distinct change in the way I felt. I had more energy, I could stay up longer, I could do more things and I felt better. After that it was more good days and fewer bad days in a steady pattern of progress. The swelling stopped being a problem.

During my semiannual visit in December of the fourth year, Dr. Brown came into my room at the hospital and told me he had a Christmas present for me. He held up the test results he had just gotten back from the laboratory, and for the first time since I had been diagnosed with scleroderma, they were negative. The disease I had been told would kill me—that kills everyone who catches it—was in remission. More than that, it had reversed.

I am very grateful for what Dr. Brown has done, and I am also grateful to the doctor who brought us together—that he cared enough about me to be open-minded and willing to believe that someone else might have the answer when he and others did not. I have talked with a lot of people with scleroderma and arthritis and other connective-tissue diseases since then, and I know that not every doctor in America is that generous.

In the several years since that happy Christmas, my test results have remained absolutely normal, with no sign of the disease. It is now ten years since I was first diagnosed, and I have reached the limit of the longest possible life that someone with my original prognosis could expect to survive. The skin on my face and hands has returned to normal; the thickening and discoloration have disappeared and it has regained its original healthy elasticity. The circulation in my fingers is not all it might be, and my fingers sometimes get cold, but their full feeling has returned and there is no trace of the disease. Changes in climate or room temperature no longer bother me. I have as much energy as I had before I came down with the disease ten years ago. I walk three miles every day, feeling great every step of the way. I can do anything I want to do. I am fully recovered.

Just a little while ago a friend of mine discovered she had lupus. I told her to get right up to see Dr. Brown as fast as she could. She said she wanted to, but she was having a lot of trouble getting her dermatologist to send her records to the National Hospital; he said Dr. Brown was a quack. My friend told him that he had helped everyone she knew that had seen him, and that he even cured a woman who had scleroderma— referring to me, but not by name. The dermatologist laughed and said, "Nobody has ever cured scleroderma. If Dr. Brown helped your friend, then she didn't have scleroderma in the first place."

"Maybe not," my friend said, "but ten years ago you seemed to think she did. You were the one who diagnosed her."

CHAPTER 26

Doctors vs. Patients

W e had a patient a few years ago who came to us from a university town in North Carolina. Before she got to us, she had been thoroughly poisoned with gold and cortisone, neither of which had worked; we treated her with tetracycline, and she did very well. She had some damaged fingers from her earlier intense rheumatoid arthritis, and when her disease had quieted down and she was feeling in good shape, she decided the time was right to get the fingers fixed. We talked it over and agreed she should go back to her hometown where there was a good hand surgeon connected with the university's medical school. A few weeks later she returned to Washington and told me this story.

When she had arrived at the office of the hand surgeon, he said he wanted her to see the rheumatologist at the university hospital. She explained that she already had a rheumatologist, but the surgeon insisted, saying that in cases involving rheumatoid arthritis, such referrals were "a matter of routine." So she made an appointment and went to see him.

The rheumatologist was the head of his department at the medical school and a very imposing figure. He exchanged a few pleasantries with my patient, then asked her what she was doing about her arthritis. She said, "Well, I see Dr. Brown in Arlington, Virginia. Do you know him?"

The doctor said, "I've heard of him. What is he giving you?"

"Tetracycline."

The rheumatologist recoiled. "That's terrible," he said. "He shouldn't be doing that."

She said, "It saved my life. My arthritis is under control for the first time in years, I've managed to get off the gold and cortisone before they killed me, and I'm doing fine."

The rheumatologist wasn't used to working with patients who really understood the nature of their medication or had the psychological energy to fight back, and he immediately retreated.

My patient, on the other hand, recognized a very familiar situation and was angry at this attempt to manipulate her. Moreover, she was the kind of lady who couldn't resist the opportunity to drive home an important point. "You know, doctor," she said, warming to her task, "I sat in your waiting room for nearly an hour before you could see me, and I had a chance to talk with a good number of your patients, most of whom tell me they have been coming to you for several years. I asked them the same question you just asked me: What are they doing about their disease? And they told me they are taking gold and cortisone. And do you know what impressed me most about those patients, Doctor? I don't believe I have ever seen such a gloomy, depressed, forlorn, and unhappy group of people in my entire life."

The doctor cleared his throat, probably in preparation to offer some kind of rejoinder, but my patient stood up cheerfully and extended her hand in farewell. "Goodness me, look at the time. I have a dinner date tonight with the chancellor of the university, and I have to run."

That was the coup de grace, and the doctor could barely rise to his feet. Somehow, he found the presence of mind to say, before she swept from the room, that he would like to see her one more time the following day. She very graciously agreed and they set the hour.

The next morning she kept her appointment, and unlike the day before the doctor saw her at precisely the specified time. His tone had changed remarkably. "I have been thinking about this all night," he said. "I believe you're doing very well with the treatment you're now getting, and I want to encourage you to keep it up."

The hand surgery went very well, and she is now free of arthritis and no longer takes medication of any kind.

IT'S NOT EASY BEING A RHEUMATOLOGIST

Doctors don't like patients who complain, and they don't like them sitting out there in the waiting room, advertisements for failure. In the field of arthritis, a subtle antagonism has developed between many doctors and their patients because of this, more than in any other field of medicine. It is not at all uncommon for patients to tell me that their previous doctor has said, "Your problem is that you can't take pain," or "It's a shame you can't take my medicine, which has been so helpful to others," or in some other way admonished them to stand up to the disease and learn to live with it. Of the 37 million stories of arthritis in America today, there are precious few in which the physician is willing to predict a happy ending. What they forecast instead, in many cases, is a gradual process of deterioration that will end in a wheelchair or a bed, with a great deal of pain.

If that situation makes the doctors angry, it makes the patients even madder. I asked one patient, from Huntsville, Alabama, why she had left her previous doctor. "Well, he had tried everything else and none of it worked," she said, "and so one day he told me he was going to try methotrexate. I'd heard that methotrexate was dangerous, and so I asked him the simple, obvious question: What had his experience been with risks from this drug? And he was so offended that he stood up, threw a syringe at me, and walked out. I walked out, too, and don't plan to go back."

It isn't uncommon for a doctor in this field to shed the patients that are difficult to deal with or who otherwise give him trouble, at the same time as he tries to collect well-to-do patients and stay as far as possible from anyone who looks like Medicare or Medicaid. The arthritics of the country aren't getting a fair shake. The rheumatology profession is one of weeding out: when a drug isn't working well or the patient is becoming more and more difficult to treat, the doctor would just as soon see him or her go someplace else.

THE SPIDERWEB

Rheumatology is a branch of medicine that works on the principle of the spiderweb. The specialist sits in the middle of the web, waiting for the general practitioners in his area to refer patients. It is a delicate art, because during this same process, the impression is created in the community that the general practitioner isn't good enough to treat arthritis.

Once the patient arrives in the rheumatologist's office, a course of treatment begins, usually with aspirin, then the nonsteroidal anti-inflammatory drugs and things of that sort. When they run out, then the patient is moved on to gold, Plaquenil, and penicillamine, and finally the immunosuppressive drugs such as Imuran and methotrexate. The whole procedure takes from two to five years, and then the point is reached where nothing works. When that finally happens, some rheumatologists simply roll over their list and send their patients back to the family practitioners who referred them in the first place. The standard phrase they use at this point is, "I'm sorry, but you can't take my medicines." It subtly places the responsibility back on the patient. And it is designed to create the impression that each patient who arrives at that condition is the only one it ever happened to, that he or she is hopelessly different. In fact, this may be the one respect in which every rheumatoid arthritic is the same: sooner or later, they all run out of medicine that works—if they live long enough—unless their physician puts them on a regimen of treatment that addresses the cause of their illness.

And this rollover process is going to continue until that happens.

One reason it may happen soon is Lyme disease.

Lyme disease looks a lot like rheumatoid arthritis. Unlike rheumatoid arthritis, however, there is a general agreement about its cause, and as a result, less than twenty years after it was first diagnosed Lyme disease now has a cure. And there is a feeling in the air that maybe rheumatoid arthritis has a knowable cause as well.

The road back has been defined, and it lies clearly before us.

Hal Roth,
now age seventy-five, was diagnosed with RA in 1991, four years after Dr. Brown's death. A friend lent him a copy of *The Road Back*, and he found a local physician to administer the therapy. Retired, he summers in Weaverville, N.C., and winters in Nokomis, Fla.

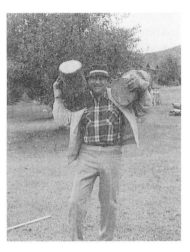

The pain started in my ankles, then migrated to my wrists and eventually moved all over my body. Walking became a problem, and climbing stairs was a challenge. Eventually I couldn't even get a good night's sleep, and I spent many nights in a reclining chair just to get some rest.

Now that's all behind me. I go up and down stairs in all confidence, walk three miles every day without a limp, and my wife and I square dance with friends for three hours at a stretch. Thank God for Dr. Brown's insight, persistence, and compassion. I wish he were still alive to see the inevitable fruit of his vision.

Kathy Schultenover
of Ohio was diagnosed with lupus in 1975. Over the next fourteen years she went through all the standard drugs from plaquenil and prednisone to methotrexate, and doctors even tried nitrogen mustard. Nothing helped. Surgery failed to close her skin ulcers, one of which was so large it threatened to expose the bone. Beginning to lose circulation, she was forced to keep her legs elevated and was no longer able to work.

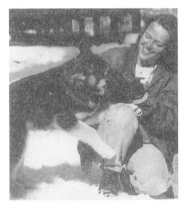

Kathy began antibiotic therapy in late 1989. Four years later her blood work was returning to normal and she was in control of her disease. That summer she took a rigorous, weeklong canoe trip of the Minnesota boundary waters with her husband and children, including portaging the boats, tents, and heavy packs. Today, with three children in college, she manages a greenhouse near the family home in Loudonville, Ohio. *Photo courtesy Columbus Dispatch*

CHAPTER 27

John Sinnott, D.O., Ida Grove, Iowa

I first came in contact with Dr. Brown's treatment several years ago through the family of a young arthritis patient here in Iowa named Don Knop. Don's folks were in the cattle business, and they heard about Dr. Brown from a woman they knew from somewhere down south who had been successfully treated by him. The family was weighing whether to send Don to the National Hospital in Washington, and they asked for my opinion.

I had to admit I knew nothing about Dr. Brown, so they gave me some tapes and articles about his approach. Everything I heard and read about the infectious nature of arthritis made good sense to me and was consistent with the things I had observed or suspected about the disease in the course of my own practice. So I did some checking in the Washington area, and learned that Dr. Brown was very highly regarded, and I recommended to the family that they send Don out to see him.

Don got better. A lot of people around here heard about it, and they asked me to send them to Washington for the same treatment. When they went, they got better, too. In a little while, it seemed that everybody in northwest Iowa and the whole Midwest was calling me up and asking me to refer them to the National Hospital. I couldn't send people I didn't know, so the Knop family asked why I didn't invite Dr. Brown out here to talk to area doctors and tell them how they could do the same thing themselves.

He came out in the summer of 1979, which was when I met him for the first time. He told me I should use his method in my own practice. When I asked him out, I had no intention of getting into that kind of treatment myself and I didn't know if I wanted to; I wasn't sure if I could or should. But he convinced me to try it. After I proved that it could work on the patients I already had who suffered from rheumatoid arthritis, I quickly found that I couldn't deny it to the other patients who started coming to me because they had heard about my results. My practice in arthritis suddenly mushroomed.

Dr. Brown's technique has been far more successful than anything I had done previously to help patients with rheumatoid arthritis and the results are better than any I have heard about elsewhere. I am satisfied that in the course of using his method I have not caused any of my patients harm, which is one of the first things that doctors who treat patients for arthritis have to think about.

I haven't done any research on my results, but I would estimate that up to about 85 percent of the patients I have treated this way have improved substantially. The remaining 15 percent represent patients whose disease was so far advanced, so aggressive, or so stubborn that I was not able to get the results I would have liked. I have always wished I lived closer to Dr. Brown so I could see how he would have handled these cases, but of course that's why I'm treating arthritics in the first place—because we live so far from the Arthritis Institute that the patients just can't get there.

As another guess, I would conservatively estimate that I have treated around two hundred patients with Dr. Brown's technique. The tradition of rheumatoid arthritis is that it's a discouraging disease and that patients don't get over it. I practice in a part of the country where people have to travel long distances, sometimes thirty miles, just to see their family doctor. There isn't any easy way to have follow-up under those circumstances, and patients don't drive that kind of distance without a good reason. I'm always amazed, even today, when I run into patients who I haven't seen in a few years and I ask them how they're doing and they say they're just fine, that the disease hasn't given them a bit of trouble in all the time since I last saw them. If I were using any other approach, I'd be pretty sure that the reason I hadn't seen them was that the treatment had failed, and not that it was such a success.

Quite a few people come to me because they have heard I'm getting good results with arthritis, and whenever someone like that walks in I make it a point to tell them I'm not an arthritis specialist, that I'm a general practitioner. The reason I do this is to let them know this isn't a dangerous technique that only a few doctors can handle, but that it's something any family practitioner can do. I tell them that if they have something requiring a specialist they should see one, but there are times when a specialist isn't necessary and this is one of them—it's so safe, even a country doctor like myself can do it.

I wish I could say that I haven't had any bad results using this approach, but that isn't the truth. My bad results—the *only* bad results—have been that Blue Cross/Blue Shield and Medicare refuse to give any recognition to this form of treatment. That's why I've lost contact with a lot of these patients; they can't afford to come back because the payment for follow-up comes right out of their pocket, and if there's nothing wrong they don't want to pay to have me to verify that they're well.

All the patients I've treated for rheumatoid arthritis have paid out of their own pockets, but there have been a lot more who turned away because they couldn't afford it, especially if it meant going into the hospital for intravenous therapy. The ones that don't have the money have been forced to find a doctor who would treat their disease with the standard arthritis medicines—treatments that cost much more, are highly dangerous, and will eventually fail—because that's the only way they can get anything under their insurance policies. And that really bothers me.

At first, Medicare wouldn't pay for the treatment because they said the approach was experimental. I've got all the paperwork showing the results with my own patients, and I've shown them all of Dr. Brown's results as well, including published research. So then they switched over to saying it's just investigational, because it's only done in a few widely scattered places around the country and hasn't been accepted nationwide as the standard treatment. It's Catch-22.

There's nothing worse than getting hopeful telephone calls from people on Medicare who are willing to drive several hundred miles to my office so I can give them some help with the pain and suffering of their rheumatoid arthritis—and having to tell them not to come because they can't afford the cost of the hospital. I won't start treatment unless I know I can get them on intravenous therapy if they need it, and most of the really bad cases do need it. It's a situation that just has got to change.

On the other side of the coin, a lot of the people who do start treatment with me are early enough in their disease that they can get good results fast. These are frequently people who have been diagnosed by other doctors and are smart enough to read up on the standard treatments before they begin; they discover that gold can be lethal and that other standard treatments can cause blindness or death, so they call me instead. Those are the people I treat and then might not see again for a couple of years until they drop by and tell me how well they are, that the arthritis is all gone. Those are the ones that make me feel good.

I suppose that if I had never met Dr. Brown, the number of arthritics I would treat in the normal course of my practice would only be about 5 percent of the number I see now. But even today the number of my arthritic patients would be a lot higher if I didn't have to turn so many away—people who are old and who Medicare won't pay for, people who are so sick they can't get here on their own, all looking for a little hope that I can't give them.

Eventually, this will change; in fact, I have seen some interesting changes already. In the time since I started using Dr. Brown's treatment, the attitude of my peers, including area rheumatologists and orthopedists, toward his infectious theory and the use of antibiotic therapy has shifted noticeably. The jokes and the snide comments have tapered off or come to an end. Other doctors read the same literature I do, and it's becoming pretty clear that the other avenues of treatment are coming to a dead end. As that happens, acceptance of the theory of an infectious source gets greater every day.

As good as it is, I'm sure that what I'm doing today is not the final answer. Dr. Brown has done almost all the work to get us to this point, and I'm certain he agrees with me that out of that groundwork there has to be an even better way to deal with this disease, one that will put it away for good for everyone. And I think he has brought us within reach of that happening.

CHAPTER 28

Rheumatoid Arthritis and Your Family Doctor

Just a few years ago, I was invited to Sweetwater, Tennessee, to talk about rheumatoid arthritis with staff doctors from the community hospital as well as other physicians from the area. My host had been a patient at the Arthritis Institute, had done well, was a member of the board of the hospital, and was concerned that there was no program of antibiotic therapy in that part of the country. There was a pretty good turnout for the meeting, partly because I told the doctors that I would be happy to look at any of their patients that they wanted me to see after the meeting.

I was particularly pleased that many of the doctors in that session were family practitioners. These days, family practitioners are very well trained in a qualification program that involves three years of hospital work, and they are capable of doing far more for patients than the general practitioners of a generation earlier. There are three reasons I feel that family practitioners are the best source for the treatment of patients suffering from rheumatoid arthritis: they are the physicians most likely to detect the disease early; they are inclined by their training toward safe remedies; and they are in the best position to provide continuity of care.

DR. CASEY

One of the family physicians who took me up on my offer was a Dr. Robert Casey, a young physician starting in family practice. After the general meeting we went to his clinic and he introduced me to a young farmer who had rheumatoid arthritis. I learned that the patient was about thirty, had a wife and four young children, and ran a successful farm in a nearby community. When I questioned him, the farmer told me he was ready to give up, and it was clear that he was terribly despondent.

He told me he had been to visit a rheumatologist in Knoxville, and that he had been on various remedies that had each, successively, failed to hold up and had made him sick. He said he was weak and tired, and that the strength had left his hands. As a farmer he needed his hands for just about everything, and he had reached the point at which he couldn't even hold on to the steering wheel of his tractor because of the weakness and pain. He said he planned to sell the farm.

In addition to wanting to help the patient for his own sake, I recognized right away that the case had all the elements to make a good demonstration for the local community of how well the basic treatment approach works. In rural areas, people tend to talk more with their neighbors than in cities, and I knew that word would get around that there was a safe, simple, inexpensive treatment for rheumatoid arthritis that really cured the disease.

Dr. Casey knew nothing more about the treatment than he had learned at our session earlier that same day, and because I worked miles away from Tennessee we all knew that I would not be available for future meetings with his patient. That was another positive aspect of this case as a model; it would be obvious to all the other physicians in the area that I wasn't stacking the deck by picking a doctor who knew everything I knew about rheumatoid arthritis and mycoplasmas. I told Dr. Casey and his patient about my plan, and they both agreed to give it a try.

I outlined a method of treatment, which included Dr. Casey calling me every couple of weeks to advise me on the patient's progress. I told the patient that he would have to hang in there for about six months, and that he would have very little encouragement during that period to indicate that good things were happening; he wouldn't feel much better, and he would still have the pain and weakness in his joints. It was a severe case. I asked, "Are you willing to fight a long battle if you know that there will be some signs of hope at the end of six months?"

He thought about it for a while, then said he would.

I also told him to find somebody in the neighborhood to give him some help with his work, that above all else he should keep the farm. "It's your livelihood, it's your future, and it's your family's future," I said. "You've got to hang on to it."

He agreed to that as well.

We started him on the program, which included some intravenous treatment to speed up the process. I no longer recall the details, but most likely it involved 250 milligrams of oral tetracycline three times a week, along with some low levels of anti-inflammatory drugs to relieve the pain, supplemented with an intravenous drip of tetracycline once every two weeks during his regular clinic visits.

As the weeks went on, Dr. Casey reported to me periodically that the patient seemed to be improving, after an initial worsening of symptoms. I asked about his spirits, which had previously been very depressed, and Casey said he thought they were picking up as well. There may have been some small adjustments to the treatment as it went along—if so, I no longer recall them—but at the end of six months Dr. Casey reported to me that the patient was almost completely well.

One of the reasons that the recovery was so dramatic is that men respond to treatment more quickly than women do. I have no idea why. Although there are exceptions on both sides, as a rule even the worst cases of rheumatoid arthritis in men show great progress in six months, and it takes women with the same degree of involvement about a third to half again as long to get to the same point. However, the difference between the sexes is not as important a factor as the length of time the patients have had the infection; the longer they have suffered from it and the more therapeutic failures they have had, the longer the time to get rid of it. There are so many other variables that I can seldom be certain just how long treatment will take, and I never promise the patient a final result by a given date. I tell them instead, "I know you are going to be all right eventually, but I don't know how long that is. Are you willing to go down this road?"

The time factor is an important consideration in starting a patient on antibiotic therapy, and it has to be handled properly at the beginning of treatment. Some doctors are concerned that they will lose their patients unless they can produce some results right away. This is the worst possible strategy: to risk the patient's well-being or even his life in exchange for short-term results. It has been my experience that when the timing is explained realistically, the patient is glad to make a commitment and stick with it to reach the sought-for remission.

As a result of his success with the young farmer, Dr. Casey decided to come to Arlington and spend a week with me at the Arthritis Institute. In the meantime, the farmer himself had been telling everyone who would listen how great the treatment was and how it had improved his life. Dr. Casey went back to Tennessee with a lot more specialized experience in treating the disease, and the Sweetwater Hospital set aside a section just for his use in working with rheumatoid arthritics.

By now Dr. Casey was getting a lot of referrals and repeating his success with arthritics from all over that part of Tennessee. He told me he had some misgivings about whether a family practitioner should be treating such a specialized practice, so with my encouragement he contacted leaders within the state Academy of Family Practice as well as educators in the discipline, including his former department head at the teaching hospital in Knoxville where he had completed his residency. He posed the question of whether it was an appropriate thing for him to be doing. Everyone he contacted told him they thought is was just fine, that the only criterion was whether the patients were achieving good results with little risk. I was impressed with that response; clearly, it put the needs of the patient first.

TETRACYCLINE THERAPY IS ABSOLUTELY SAFE

The reason I was able to work with Dr. Casey—and over the years with many other doctors who were a long distance away and whose patients I never met—was that we were dealing with a treatment that was absolutely safe. Tetracycline has been used for a long time in two chronic conditions without ill effect: bronchiectasis in old people and acne in the young. It would have been impossible to do this same thing with any of the kinds of therapy that are usually prescribed for rheumatoid arthritis, because they involve such substantial risk to the patient. At the outset, the process requires explanation and it needs guidance. Dr. Casey got to the point where he had a real instinct for the mechanism, and from there on he didn't need any further help.

Some patients are more sensitive than others to medication, and part of learning how to work with tetracycline is developing a reliable feel for how much is right in each case. This is made much easier by the fact that the dosage level which a patient accepts best is also the level that works best therapeutically; it isn't a matter of sensitive patients missing a part of the benefits because they need more tetracycline than they can handle.

Patients who react poorly to one form of tetracycline will frequently respond well to another. It is a drug that has been around long enough to be available in lots of forms. We have found, for example, that patients who do not respond well to tetracycline are often favorably responsive to oxytetracycline, a compound that is nearly identical chemically, or the other mycin drugs such as erythromycin, Vibramycin, or clindamycin. If there is a strong streptococcal history or a high level of antibodies against the streptococcus, ampicillin may have to be introduced. The main point is for the physician to gain a complete understanding of this mechanistic approach to guide his individualized strategy through the shifting terrain of rheumatoid arthritis. The doctor has to recognize that he is dealing with a very delicately balanced condition. It is a lot like walking through the woods in the dark; if you're on familiar ground and can recognize the landmarks as they pass underfoot, you get where you want to go—and if you miss, you run into the trees.

One of the problems with arthritis is that many of its victims can't tolerate any kind of oral medicine because their stomachs have become extremely reactive through long and escalating sensitization from many different medicines. Patients who may experience upset from taking tetracycline orally are likely to find that they have no such reaction when they start taking it intravenously. A third choice is intramuscular injection in the form of clindamycin; it is somewhat less effective than intravenous, but it's an alternative for patients whose blood vessels are hard to reach. (Someday, I expect we will see an antimycoplasma medication in a form that can be administered rectally, so it goes directly into the bloodstream without aggravating the oversensitized stomach.)

Family physicians are no strangers to monitoring and managing these kinds of variables as they treat the entire range of health problems they face daily. In most cases, they quickly master the subtleties of finding the most effective combination of form, dosage, and methodology for successful antibiotic therapy. They are careful not to use dangerous drugs. A busy practitioner simply does not have the time to monitor risky medications. Until now, the rheumatologist's role was essentially to guard against kidney, retinal, bone marrow, liver, and lung damage. The requirements of his vigil narrowed down the likelihood of reaching more than a handful of the 37 million arthritics in our country. With a safer method

CHAPTER 29

Hon. Thomas C. Reed

After serving as secretary of the Air Force during the Ford Administration, I returned to my construction and land development business in the spring of 1977—and in transit I took a long skiing vacation in Breckenridge, Colorado. During that vacation, I hurt my shoulder in a fall.

I didn't pay much attention to it at first; it was sore but not particularly painful, and I expected it would take care of itself as those things do. I was in my mid-forties, and when the soreness persisted, I assumed it just meant I had reached an age when that kind of thing takes a little longer. But it got steadily worse.

That summer I took my family out to our house in California. I like to swim, but every time I got into our pool the pain in my shoulder was more severe than the last, and I finally decided to give in to it and see about getting it fixed.

I went to our family doctor. I've always liked him; he's good at spotting problems, he isn't someone who makes a big deal out of a little one, and he has a good record for getting me back on my feet fast. He examined me thoroughly and said I probably had a touch of something like bursitis—but that what it really came down to was simply that I was getting older. If you have that kind of a fall in your mid-forties, you don't expect to bounce the way you did when you were twenty. He told me to let nature take care of it, and in the meantime to be careful not to do anything that might hurt the shoulder further. He also said I might eventually want a shot of cortisone, and he gave me the names of a couple of rheumatologists if the problem continued to get worse.

The problem did continue to get worse, but I was extremely busy and didn't take the time to do anything further about it for another several months. By that fall it had become very difficult for me to lift my arms over my head to put on a sweater, take a shower, or do anything else that required that kind of motion. It also slowed me down at work. I was trying to pick up my business again after working for the government, and I found myself hurting every time I reached up to get something out of a file. Business trips were a big part of my life, and they became an ordeal in which I knew I would have to endure several hours of aches, twinges, and stiffness.

In early November I spoke about it with my uncle Lawrence Reed, and he recommended that I see Dr. Brown over at the National Hospital.

Probably the thing that decided me was a trip we had scheduled with the kids. We had chartered a boat in the Caribbean for the Thanksgiving vacation, and as I looked forward to it I kept thinking how difficult it was going to be for me to swim and dive and do the other things we usually did on those trips with my shoulder in that condition. I gave Dr. Brown a call and went over to see him.

He had ordered some blood tests first, so by the time I got to meet him he already knew what was going on and was able to tell me exactly where I stood. He said I had tested positive for rheumatoid arthritis and that the trouble I was having with my shoulder wasn't going to get better if I continued to ignore it.

He told me what was involved in the disease—what causes it and how it can be successfully treated—and I have to admit that I learned more about mycoplasmas that day than I really wanted to know. My immediate purpose in going to him was to get fixed up so I could go sailing. I had no idea before then what a truly terrible disease rheumatoid arthritis can be.

Dr. Brown also told me about depression—that it was as much a part of rheumatoid arthritis as the pains and stiffness, and that it would go away with the rest of the symptoms as a result of his treatment. That wasn't something I had discussed with anyone else, but I was certainly aware that my spirits had been low as a result of the problem in my shoulder.

He started me off on aspirin to reduce the pain, along with intravenous treatments with an antibiotic, a form of tetracycline. He also told me that I wasn't going to be immediately better as a result of the treatment, and certainly not in time to get rid of the pain before I went sailing. He said it would be a gradual process, but that one day I would notice that it was starting to improve.

I remember Dr. Brown telling me that, because that's pretty much how it turned out. There was a total of about five intravenous treatments, spaced progressively further apart for a period of perhaps five months, along with daily doses of Clinoril (a nonsteroidal anti-inflammatory) and a couple of tetracycline tablets twice a week. I did go sailing with the family as planned, but as far as the arthritis was concerned it was an ordeal.

One day after about five months I was in the shower and when I reached up to get something, I realized the pain was completely gone. I said to myself, "It's all over. Amazing." I used up the rest of the pills Dr. Brown had given me but didn't bother to refill the prescription.

Things went along fine for a couple of years. In 1983, I began to get some of the familiar aches, stiffness, and twinges.

It wasn't as serious as the first incidence of arthritis, but once you've been hit between the eyes by a two-by-four, you look twice when you see someone down the street holding the same kind of board. So I headed right back to Dr. Brown. He did the usual blood tests and started me on the pills again. This time the arthritis went away in less than eight weeks.

Despite the fact that I can remember a particular event that made me aware my arthritis had left me the first time, I know that isn't the way the disease usually ends. It isn't like a bell going off to let you out of class or a tooth being pulled that cures the toothache. But there are moments—and they recur more frequently as you keep improving—when you realize you have regained your cheerful outlook on life, when you can pour a cup of coffee without getting a pain in your wrist and you can take a normal shower. Eventually those moments become continuous, and you realize it's over.

For the past three years I have taken no medication whatever and have remained totally free of any symptoms of rheumatoid arthritis. My energy level is as high as it has ever been, my spirits are up where they should be, I can travel without stiffness, swim without pain, and lead a normal life that is full and productive. Dr. Brown describes this as remission, because that's how doctors talk about a good result.

I call it a cure.

How Tetracycline Works

When I first started working on rheumatoid arthritis at the Rockefeller Institute in the late 1930s, I decided to retrace a path that had been well worn by earlier investigators; I went to the joint fluid, looking for any signs of an infectious agent.

It was already established that regular bacteria don't operate in those parts of the body; such bacteria are hard to miss, and hundreds of earlier investigators had failed to isolate any infectious agent from the joint fluid of an arthritic. That didn't rule out regular bacteria as causative factors, but if streptococci were involved, for example, they apparently worked by setting up a command post elsewhere in the body—in a gland, probably—and telegraphing their effects, via toxins, to the afflicted areas. What I was looking for was some smaller organism, closer to the size of a virus, that lived and worked right in the joint.

SABIN'S MOUSE

It happened that Albert Sabin was working in a laboratory just down the hall at the time, studying a central nervous system disease called toxoplasmosis. One day he told me he had cultured the brain of a mouse and come up with a strain of mycoplasma. He said he nearly missed it; when he smeared the culture out and tried to stain it, he couldn't see anything, but something was clouding the media and he knew that some kind of organism was growing there. When he finally identified it as a mycoplasma, he put some of the cloudy culture fluid in a hypodermic and injected another mouse. As a result, the second mouse came down with a case of arthritis.

At the same time, I had succeeded in isolating a mycoplasma organism from the joint fluid of a human. For some reason, it was much more difficult to work with than was the mouse strain of mycoplasma. In later years, our work with gorillas and elephants would support those early observations that the mycoplasma strains associated with more complex immune systems in the higher animals are more difficult to isolate and study, although exactly why is still unknown.

The main area from which it was possible to recover mycoplasmas was the genital tract. When I got back to Johns Hopkins, I worked with specialists there and got cultures from the cervix in females and prostatic secretions in men, cultured them, and found mycoplasmas. Those strains had in common with the strains from Sabin's mouse cultures that they were susceptible to the same gold and quinine drugs that have an effect on arthritis. There was an obvious connection between mycoplasmas and arthritis in humans, just as Sabin had found there was in mice.

LOOKING FOR LOW-RISK ALTERNATIVES

Because the long-term risks were so much more substantial than any short-term benefits, I didn't want to use gold or Plaquenil to treat my arthritis patients. I started looking at all sorts of antibiotics for alternatives. Working with a brilliant, enthusiastic research fellow from Harvard named Jack Nunemaker whom the head of my department at Hopkins assigned to my project, I soon found there was one class of antibiotics that worked on mycoplasmas, and that was tetracycline, the so-called mycin group. The group included Aureomycin, Terramycin, Achromycin, lincomycin, erythromycin, Vibramycin, and clindamycin.

If mycoplasmas were difficult to isolate, in theory they would be even more difficult to eradicate, since they were either intercellular or under a great deal of inflammatory tissue. Because of that difficulty, I had no hesitancy about relentlessly pursuing the treatment with Aureomycin. If one were to think of rheumatoid arthritis as an ordinary infection, common sense would say to quit treatment if the patient didn't become well within a few days. But if the disease were viewed instead as a bacterial allergy, common sense would say to persist. That recognition of the true nature of the disease was an important turning point in understanding how it could eventually be subdued.

TETRACYCLINE IS NOT LIKE OTHER ANTIBIOTICS

The persistent use of tetracycline in pursuit of an infectious allergy ran against the common view of how antibiotics should be applied. Antibiotics were generally regarded at the time as a short-term response, used to treat pneumonia, strep throat, and other bacterial disorders, and were never used over an extended period because of the risk that the patients would develop immune strains of the germ for which they were being treated. This view was softened somewhat in more recent years by the discovery that some problems, particularly acne in children and bronchiectasis, a chronic affliction of older people marked by paroxysmic coughing, could only be cured by using antibiotics for a long time. But generally the expectation remains that antibiotics should produce results quickly, and if they don't, then the doctor should try something else.

TETRACYCLINE DOES NOT GIVE RISE TO IMMUNE STRAINS OF GERMS

The prolonged use of most antibiotics can indeed give eventual rise to an immune strain of germ. Immunity is developed in a germ's outer surface, which is the area affected by penicillin and other antibiotics. Tetracycline is different from all other antibiotics in that critical respect: it affects the core of the germ, not the outer surface, and therefore no immune strain of germs ever develops as a result of its use. Moreover, people who use tetracycline over a period of months or years tend to avoid colds, pneumonia, and other diseases.

Once the view of arthritis as an infectious allergy relieved us of the pressure for those immediate results, we were able to shift our attention to various manipulative techniques for increasing its effectiveness under varying conditions. Oral treatment worked just fine in relatively early cases, for example, where the degree of inflammatory reaction or obstruction by scar tissue had not had the opportunity to build up; longer-standing cases responded far better to intravenous treatment. These facts, too, supported the concept of the mechanism as we were coming to understand it.

GETTING WORSE, THEN GETTING BETTER

The Herxheimer phenomenon was further evidence that rheumatoid arthritis involved the release of an antigen or toxin rather than the more common disease process of a broad-scale bacterial invasion. I noticed in the beginning that when treatment was started with antibiotics, as many as 80 percent of the recipients got worse before they got better, indicating that the treatment was hitting a susceptible source.

It is interesting to note that the Herxheimer effect does not occur when one is treating a streptococcal infection with a penicillin derivative. The streptococcus is not located at the site of the irritation, is not protected by a barrier of inflamed or scarred tissue, and it is knocked out in the faster, more conventional manner of regular bacterial infections.

We know that tetracycline works on mycoplasmas specifically, and to a lesser extent on streptococci, but doesn't have a particular effect on other bacteria. Further, conventional bacteria would not be controllable by any antibiotic that was administered intravenously only once every two weeks or once a month. The reason for that broad period with tetracycline is to avoid a build-up of sensitivity to the drug so the body won't block its action against the mycoplasmas.

Because the process is a bacterial allergy, this approach works very well. By contrast, treatment of pneumonia with an antibiotic requires a round-the-clock assault on the pneumococcus germ in order to keep it suppressed until the body can take over and get rid of it; in that case, treatments spaced two weeks apart would simply allow the bacteria to build up again and come back stronger than ever. With a bacterial allergy, by contrast, the germ creates a little wall around itself, a tiny zone of toxin, which keeps the disease-fighting antibodies from reaching it; the therapeutic approach with tetracycline is simply to suppress the toxin, which is the germ's means of defense. The fact that tetracycline works in precisely that manner when used on rheumatoid arthritis is further proof of the infectious nature of the disease; if therapy is administered intermittently or unevenly, the results are intermittent or uneven in the same pattern. The same logic that linked mycoplasmas with arthritis in Sabin's mouse also proves the presence of mycoplasmas in humans when tetracycline is used as a therapeutic probe.

When tetracycline is used to suppress the toxin, the disease is eventually driven into remission. When it is not, the toxin enables the germ to stay in its host for twenty, forty, or sixty years—unless, of course, the host succumbs in the interim to some other form of treatment.

CHAPTER 31

A Physician's Guide to the Use of Tetracycline in Rheumatoid Arthritis

When a doctor starts any course of treatment that affects the antigen of this disease, he has to keep in mind that the tissues of the arthritic are very reactive and do not like medicines very much—but neither do they require much. The doctor also has to keep in mind a conceptual view of the disease process during treatment. An early case will accept medicine much better than a late one. A case in which the rheumatoid factor is negative is very much easier to treat than one in which it is positive. In either case, treatment cannot begin by throwing the book at a patient. Generally it starts by giving medication twice a week.

The allergic state in itself is anti-germ. This is an extremely important point. Sir William Osler, the great physician-in-chief at the Johns Hopkins Medical School at the turn of the century, observed that asthmatics were immune to getting pneumonia. He based that conclusion on the terrible epidemic in Philadelphia in which around a third of the population died of lobar pneumonia; the asthmatics came through that epidemic scot-free, although one might reasonably have expected that they would be among the first to go. When I was at Johns Hopkins some years later, I heard of Osler's observation and it amazed me. I tried to understand why that could be the case.

When the opportunity presented itself, I got some sputum from an asthmatic and looked at it for bacteria. Under the microscope it appeared to be sterile. I got some cultures, and nothing grew. Osler had been right; there is something in the asthmatic's system that is anti-germ.

I tried to imagine what it could be. We knew that asthmatics produce histamine, which causes the bronchial tree to go into spasms. The histamine figures in an allergic reaction which is very delicately poised; pollen or some other irritant comes along and the muscles in the bronchial tubes squeeze down and contract. But that didn't explain the sterility. I filed the phenomenon away in my mind and went on to other things.

When I started in arthritis research at the Rockefeller Institute, the clinical side of the institute was a hospital for special diseases. I took care of a ward in the institute hospital that was filled with children with rheumatic fever. We knew that rheumatic fever was due to streptococcus; the first person to type out the streptococcus was Rebecca Lansfield, who was at the Institute at that time. One of the most vicious forms was Type A, and that was the one that showed up most often in rheumatic fever.

Children who had had rheumatic fever were on the hospital's list, so every time one of them got another attack—and recurrence was a common feature of the disease in those days—the child would be rushed right back to the hospital, where I would do an immediate throat culture and try to grow the strep. But I found that by the time they got there with their disease, the strep was gone from their throats.

It didn't make any sense. At first I thought that maybe I didn't know how to culture it, so I sought out an ear, nose and throat specialist and went through the procedure in detail to be sure I was doing it right. Then, on a hunch, we changed the timing of our studies, advising the parents on our list to bring their children into the hospital as soon as they got a sore throat, and not to wait for the rheumatic fever attack that generally ensued. I did throat cultures on those children when they arrived, and the Type A streptococcus grew easily. But as I continued the cultures over the next couple of weeks, by the time the inflammation and joint swelling appeared, the strep had gone away. We knew that the tonsils were still infected, but that was under the surface.

It dawned on me that this was the same thing that Osler had noticed with asthma. Any allergic state created by any cause—pollen, or by the germ itself—would drive the germ out of sight. The bacterial allergy of rheumatic fever had driven away the streptococcus that created the allergy. This realization was tremendously illuminating: I realized that it wasn't necessary to be able to see the germ in order to have the condition. It is reassuring to be able to culture the organism that is creating a condition, but the inability to culture it in no way means that the germ isn't still there, in hiding.

When penicillin came along and was proven to have a killing effect on the streptococcus, it wiped out rheumatic fever.

When I returned to Johns Hopkins, I began to think about the implications of this insight about allergy as it related to other diseases. I knew that undulant fever, for example, was commonly transmitted by the bodies of diseased animals to slaughterhouse workers, but that it had never been shown to be transmitted from one human to another. The reason for this had to be that the allergic response in humans was driving the brucella underground and sterilizing the surfaces in just the same way that rheumatic fever sterilized the surfaces of streptococci.

Eventually, I realized that the same process was going on in rheumatoid arthritis, and just because we couldn't see the mycoplasma, there was no reason to believe it wasn't still there, causing the trouble. That also explained the great difficulty we were having in growing mycoplasma in a culture medium. It was highly allergy-producing, it sensitized the host, and the allergic reaction was covering it up. In effect, mycoplasma planted a forest and then hid among the trees. But we realized that this same forest was also protecting the host from an unwelcome intruder. The conventional view of allergies as a mean twist in the immune system causing something to go awry was no longer quite as valid. Nature put the allergic reaction in place in order to isolate the disease source and keep it from spreading. It happens to give symptoms, but there is a reason for it. I remembered a comment by one of my early teachers, Dr. William Tillett, who told me that in order to understand disease it was necessary to take a germ's-eye view.

For his illustration of how the germ sees things, Dr. Tillett invited me to consider why the pneumococcus germ chooses the lung as the place to live out its life, or why the meningococcus selects the meninges that surround the brain, or why the poliovirus picks one small cell in the spinal column to do its work and nowhere else, or why the typhoid bacillus chooses a small lymphoid patch in the intestinal tract from which to go out and do all its dirty work in the body. I said, "I suppose it's because those diseases find some kind of enzyme systems in those places that supports their lives, and they can't find those enzymes anywhere else."

"I think you've got it," Dr. Tillett said.

When I found that mycoplasmas had an attraction for the synovium and for the lung and the genital tract, I assumed it was because there was something present in those areas which would support them—in some cases for years. With mycoplasmas, we need further research to determine what that source of special attraction might be.

As for the significance of our understanding of the allergic state, we know that it serves a useful purpose in keeping the germ from spreading, but it doesn't stop it from producing toxins to which the body can become allergic and which then produce disease. We also know that if the treatment neutralizes those toxins that keep the germ localized—by using cortisone or too much anti-inflammatory medication—and doesn't go for their source, then all the treatment does is deprive the body of its one natural defense, letting the cat out of the bag. That process characterizes the typical course of conventional arthritis treatment: great quantities of pain-relievers, most of which are anti-inflammatory, give momentary symptomatic remission at the same time as they allow the disease to spread. And when they fail, they fail terribly.

At one time, the principal anti-inflammatory was cortisone. I recall one patient who came to me with a terrific cortisone dependency. Her previous doctors couldn't get the dosage level down, and she began to get sick from the cortisone effect, developing an ulcer in the gastrointestinal tract, hemorrhages, and other problems. The reason they couldn't lower the cortisone was that by then the cat was out of the bag and they were trying to use the same drug that had released it to block the pain produced everywhere in her body. Even to reduce her daily dose from fifty milligrams to forty-nine produced terrible pain. When she arrived at the Institute, we went for the source of the problem with intravenous tetracycline to attack the mycoplasma directly. Simply by suppressing the antigen in this manner, within three weeks we were able to reduce her cortisone requirement by 80 percent.

These days, most doctors are really afraid of cortisone, and they often go to extremes to avoid using it at all. I have never had a fear of cortisone in small doses and I frequently use it to deal with the inflammation while I attack the source of the antigen with antibiotics. The danger is not in using cortisone as a palliative, but rather in relying on it as the primary therapeutic weapon; the requirement is bound to keep mounting as the antigen, which it ignores, is allowed to increase unchecked.

The only acceptable excuse for liberating antigen in a rheumatoid arthritic is to kill its source.

To that end, we start off a typical patient with tetracycline three times a week, usually on Monday, Wednesday, and Friday. The drug is not manufactured in units less than 250 milligrams, although at one time I had it made up in

10-milligram amounts and gradually increased it to avoid the Herxheimer reaction. Nowadays we start off with the 250 milligrams, letting the Herxheimer effect occur and then treating it with symptomatic remedies.

People vary enormously in the anti-inflammatory drugs which they can use during this stage of treatment. We often start with aspirin, but we also use a wide variety of substitutes for cortisone—and sometimes small doses of the cortisone itself (one to five milligrams of prednisone a day, for example, but never more than ten and preferably none) to block the inflammatory reaction. We are careful to keep the doses of any of these drugs low enough that we don't interfere with the immune system, but rather just deal with the allergy.

An interesting thing happens to people who have a lot of regular allergies such as hay fever and skin eruptions and who start treatment for the bacterial allergy of rheumatoid arthritis: the regular allergies often get better. This points to the possibility that bacterial allergies may be one of the pacesetters for the general allergic state. I suspect that to be the case: that there is a primary allergen which in many instances comes from bacteria, and that it is added to by feathers, dust, pollen, and other irritants, and that those outside sources, long regarded as primary, may in fact be secondary.

As the treatment progresses, the doctor gradually increases the amount of antibiotic. There are lots of ways to do this: it can move up to 250 milligrams twice a day two days a week; twice a day three times a week; or a larger dosage on the original schedule of once a day three times a week. Care has to be taken not to go so high that the treatment triggers an allergic reaction; arthritics are so sensitized that they can become allergic to just about anything, including medicines that don't normally cause much allergy. The most I would prescribe orally would be 500 milligrams three times a day on Monday and Friday.

If the patient doesn't respond as well as I'd like to oral medication, I administer the drug intravenously. Recently I saw a patient who came up from Ecuador, and she had been treated with every drug available—cortisone, gold, Plaquenil, chloroquine—and had not only become refractory to each of those forms of medicine but was getting steadily and predictably worse. Moreover, it was virtually impossible to treat her with oral medicines because she had built up a resistance to practically everything. I treated her intravenously with tetracycline and a fair amount of pain-relieving anti-inflammatory medicine, and she did very well. She was not particularly exceptional; a lot of the patients we get have been so badly overmedicated that the stomach reacts to almost any medicine we put in it and we have to treat them by injection.

Regardless of how badly a patient has been sensitized to medicines, either from prior medication or from the disease itself, there is almost always some way to get around an adverse reaction until the system is back in sufficient balance to accept medication without adverse effects.

Not all of the standard treatments run out of steam after the same length of time. Gold tends to work for quite a while, often two years and sometimes longer, before it folds up. Once the patient gets sensitized to the first of these substances, however, the next ones to come along don't hold up for quite as long; either the drug loses its initial beneficial effect in a shorter time or the drug starts to produce other effects, such as skin eruptions, and treatment has to be stopped. All other things being equal, the standard drug which the patient can usually tolerate the longest is gold, followed by Plaquenil and then penicillamine. As noted repeatedly in this book, the basic problem with every one of these drugs is that each is extremely dangerous in its own right, regardless of the effects it may have on the process of sensitization; each can be lethal.

Very difficult cases of sensitization require a certain amount of persistence in seeking the right combination of antibiotic dosage and method of administration. And it is not possible to overstate the necessity for caution in the use of cortisone, which in excessive quantities can interfere with the body's defenses. The defense mechanism and the allergic mechanism are tied together in a way; an allergy is itself a form of defense and plays a role in keeping germs suppressed; on another level, the antibody seems to attach itself to the organism, making it possible for the white blood cell to become active in destroying the germ. If too much cortisone is given, that second level of defense is blocked and the purpose of the primary medicine is defeated. A small amount of an anti-inflammatory drug, sometimes even cortisone, on the other hand, suppresses the inflammatory component without blocking the basic immune mechanism, allowing the antibiotic to breach the wall around the organism and do its work.

In that connection, it has been well established that when a medicine blocks a reaction, as cortisone does, and then is stopped, the result is an explosion. When a woman goes into remission during pregnancy, it is because the body is producing extra amounts of natural cortisone to block the arthritis, and when the baby is born the mother suffers a terrible rebound flare. It is particularly difficult for an arthritic mother to have to go through this painful experience right at the time she is trying to take care of her new baby. For that reason, we often hold off on anti-inflammatory medication during the period of the pregnancy, but as soon as the mother is delivered we give it to her right away in order to avoid that flare.

The length of time patients require in treatment can vary widely, depending primarily on how long they have had the disease. In the most entrenched and recalcitrant cases, it can take up to thirty months from the beginning of therapy until the patient clearly turns the corner toward improvement, and the achievement of lasting remission can take several years.

Once the blood begins to look good, the anemia is corrected, the rheumatoid factor is down, the sedimentation and hemoglobin are where they ought to be, and the mycoplasma antibodies are beginning to peter out, I know the patient is close to remission. The antibodies are probably the key indicator; they start high, rise with the Herxheimer reaction, and then begin to fall as therapy is continued. Even if the progress toward recovery should turn downward again for a short time,

PART III
PATIENTS' RIGHTS

CHAPTER 32.

The Search for Rightside Up

There are two likely explanations for why antibiotic therapy has proven so effective in treating the rheumatoid forms of arthritis and other connective tissue diseases. The more obvious rationale is Dr. Brown's still very plausible hypothesis that an infectious agent is fundamental to the onset of the disease, and perhaps even to its chronicity. But Dr. Brown was also aware that that hypothesis probably did not stand alone, and today it is coupled in all ongoing research with the fact that antibiotic therapy is also anti-inflammatory, the latter effect being independent of any antimicrobial activity. Several years ago, after reading *The Road Back*, Dr. Rothschild wrote, "This is the first time that I realized the tetracycline was being provided for its long-term impact. As tetracycline also has immunomodulatory effects, this is quite fascinating."

A number of the current therapies that are generally characterized as anti-inflammatory drugs, including steroids, methotrexate, gold, and all the standard agents that have migrated into the field of rheumatology, are equally mysterious in the way they achieved their effects. "We just don't know how they work," Dr. Trentham says. "They work partially in some patients; we can't predict in which patients they have this partial effect. Obviously they still are too toxic to be highly popular, and because of that toxicity we're still seeking alternative therapies. That's a lot of the rationale for further evaluating antibiotic therapy, because of its inherent safety, at least with the tetracycline drugs."

Meanwhile, Dr. Trentham defended the principle of using other drugs, even when it is obvious they won't affect an infectious agent, simply because they might still help the patient overall. He offered the analogy of the patient with pneumonia. It's usually a type of bacteria that causes the disease, and doctors can effectively cure pneumonia by giving penicillin, an antibiotic. But regardless of whether the patient is treated with an antibiotic at the outset, it's well established that giving aspirin will at least make the patient feel better; it doesn't get to the heart of the matter, but it still provides a benefit.

Like Tom Brown, Dr. Trentham uses cortisone very sparingly and only to the extent that it eases suffering and increases the patient's tolerance for the sometimes long period of waiting for the antibiotic therapy to show its results.

"I think there is a lot of truth in Dr. Brown's feeling that the use of steroids, overall, is not a good approach to the disease. They buy short-term efficacy, but longer exposure does lead to deleterious side effects that he was well aware of. It's a two-edged blade that we all have to play with, but he provided a real service in voicing his concern and caution.I think that today all rheumatologists appreciate that concept."

Collectively, most of those second-line agents Dr. Trentham cited are called DMARDs, an acronym for disease modifying anti-rheumatic drug; another name is slow-acting drug. With any of them, but particularly with the old standard gold, rheumatologists realized it could take six months for patients to respond, if they were going to respond at all, and during that time it was commonplace, when patients were suffering acute pain, to give them a short course of steroids for immediate help. The dosage was kept as low as possible; for most rheumatologists, the cutoff would be 10 milligrams or less of prednisone a day. However, that kind of restraint was still hardly a universal standard. As recently as 1990, a lupus sufferer in New York lost his sight to cataracts after being treated for months with prednisone in dosage levels of *twenty times* that amount.

HEREDITY REVISITED

Another development in the early '90s was the growing body of new evidence about the potential role of heredity. Tom Brown had recognized the strong hereditary predisposition to the disease, and from time to time all rheumatologists encounter striking instances in which rheumatoid arthritis permeates the family—although today most rheumatologists accept Dr. Brown's thesis that this predisposition is not the cause *per se*. Trentham chronicled one such case from his own experience.

Robert and Nancy Sawyer lived in Greenfield, Massachusetts, and by late 1992 Nancy, a travel agent, had been Trentham's patient for fifteen years. He described the entire family as being highly intelligent, motivated people.

Nancy's mother, Helen Caldwell Thayer, was born in 1894. Her husband was a doctor and, although there was always a reluctance to say she had rheumatoid arthritis, surviving family members recalled that she suffered from some form of joint disease most of her adult life. Nancy was born in 1928 and suffered from severe rheumatoid arthritis since the late 1970s, when she was almost fifty. They have four children: Amy Clark, born in 1954; Geoff, born in 1956; Martha Folsom, born in 1959; and Jenny Torgersen, born in 1963. Amy has been spared the disease, but one of her five children, Emily, was diagnosed with juvenile rheumatoid arthritis in 1989. At the time Mrs. Sawyer offered the family's medical history, Emily was thirteen and she had only been treated with aspirin. The disease wasn't at a point where her doctor wanted to risk stirring things up by using anything stronger. Nancy's son, Geoff, had been spared as well, as had his two children. Martha had rheumatoid arthritis, but no children. Jenny had it as well, although her children so far did not.

FAMILY TREE

Family members diagnosed with (or suspected of having) RA in **bold**

Helen Caldwell Thayer
1894–1954

Nancy Thayer Sawyer
1928–

Amy S. Clark	Geoff Sawyer	**Martha S. Folsom**	**Jenny S. Torgersen**
1954–	1956–	1959–	1963–
One	One		One
Emily (1977–)	Two		Two
Three			
Four			
Five			

"Of course," Mrs. Sawyer cautioned, "it would be premature to say the picture is complete: rheumatoid arthritis waited fifty years in my case, and it could take as long for any of the others. But we know it has been present in at least three generations of the family, and probably four."

SUSPECTS AND SCENARIOS

Given that hereditary liability, what happens next is still the subject of speculation and debate. One theory is that a bacterial or other infectious agent comes into the host and, because a portion of that organism has a shape similar to a tissue constituent in the joint the body first mounts an immune attack on the foreign organism that may or may not get rid of it. The attack is targeted to the structure of the invading organism, and because the structure mimics or is identical to perhaps a host protein or tissue constituent, it may be that there is then a secondary response directed against the body. This is the so-called auto-immune attack, or anti-self reactivity, in which the nature of the process turns inward and attacks the patient in a pattern that propagates rheumatoid arthritis. The theory is termed molecular mimicry. Many of these infectious agents are quite old phylogenetically, going back many millennia. These ancient, highly conserved organisms arose at a time in evolution when their structure was very close to the structure of other living organisms, including mammals.

If indeed rheumatoid arthritis is caused by such an infectious agent, there are several promising candidates. One is a tuberculosis-like organism, a mycobacterial species that still hasn't been identified but is suspected to be a cousin to the bug that causes tuberculosis. Another strong possibility is that it could be a virus, perhaps some very primitive type of retrovirus that can hide itself completely—or it could be similar to the virus that causes AIDS, which again would affect a certain cell, the T cell, and initially remain very quiet and elusive of detection. Or it still could be a mycoplasmal organism, as Tom Brown suspected. Others now suspect mycoplasmas as well. Up until very recently, however, despite Tom Brown's pioneering efforts at the Rockefeller Institute sixty years ago, mycoplasmas remained amazingly elusive to scrutiny. The wall would crack dramatically in 1995, with the breakthrough in Bordeaux (see "Evidence Accumulated," page 24).

Although mycobacteria, viruses, and mycoplasmas are the three leading infectious suspects, a fourth possibility may be nothing more complex than a fairly common bacterial invader of the sort we're all exposed to from time to time, such as a streptococcus, the organism that causes sore throats and still occasionally rheumatic fever. If that's the cause, then it would appear that only in people who are allergic or sensitive to the organism, based on their hereditary makeup, does the process go on to develop rheumatoid arthritis.

THE MYSTERIOUS ROLE OF T CELLS

Another feature of what many physicians call the second phase of this disease, frequently identified as the "auto-immune" phase, is an attack on the joints by the body's white blood cells. The original invader may or may not be present when the attack takes place, but most scientists are now convinced that the type of cell that's producing the problem in rheumatoid arthritis is indeed the T cell mentioned earlier, and it seems to be the very same T cell that becomes infected in AIDS.

The natural role of the T cell is to kill foreign cells or those that have become infected by virus. It does this by helping other cells respond to antigens, or by suppressing the activity of specific populations of cells. The role of T cells in these two diseases became dramatically apparent in those cases where a patient with rheumatoid arthritis also contracts AIDS, and the arthritis simply disappears. Conversely, in patients who already have active AIDS, their bodies are not able to generate sufficient numbers of these T cells to develop rheumatoid arthritis. This phenomenon has been under intense investigation for the better part of a decade and is now recognized throughout the world. By the time of the MIRA trial not a single case of active rheumatoid arthritis had been reported in an AIDS patient, nor had an AIDS patient been known to develop any form of the disease.

"All of this background fits very nicely into the context of Dr. Brown's thinking, and from that standpoint he really was quite provocative and innovative at the time," Dr. Trentham said. "He took it as far as he could, given the existing knowledge. AIDS did not exist when he developed his theory. There was a little bit of evidence that rheumatoid arthritis was a tuberculosis-like disease, and certainly there was a great interest in infectious-disease candidates such as mycoplasma and streptococci that continues today. But this is not a theory that died and now may be coming back to life again; it's really a logical continuum in the evolution of Dr. Brown's thinking."

Although Dr. Trentham and his coworkers were among the first to recognize the importance of the T cell in rheumatoid arthritis, he is quick to credit many other researchers for equally pivotal roles in the research that eventually produced the shift back toward the infectious theory.

The first true pioneer in the field was Harold Paulus, the UCLA rheumatologist whose editorial in *Annals of Internal*

Medicine would introduce the MIRA study in 1995. Back in the 1960s, Paulus was the first person to hook up patients with rheumatoid arthritis to a plastic tube that went into their thoracic duct, the structure in the chest where lymph first enters the blood to commence its trip throughout the body. The major cell constituent in lymph is the T cell. By eliminating these cells in the thoracic duct, Paulus made the striking observation that patients with rheumatoid arthritis would get remarkably better within two or three days after starting this intervention, and they stayed better as long as this tube continued to drain their lymph.

This avenue of research received another major boost some years later when Dr. van Boxel of the NIH first reported that almost all the cells in the joints in rheumatoid arthritis were T cells.

In about 1981, a group at Harvard headed by Trentham and another group at Stanford Medical School led by Dr. Samuel Strober, both showed that one could treat rheumatoid arthritis using a radiation therapy technique identical to that developed to combat Hodgkin's disease, a lymphatic cancer. Because Hodgkin's also triggers the production of T cells, and since patients improved after radiation therapy, it became all the more plausible that the T cell was indeed central to the disease. This research in radiation therapy may also have given an unintended boost to the popularity of exposure to radon gas and visits to abandoned uranium mines, a folk remedy among arthritis sufferers in the Southwest. For many years, mild radiation has also been an accepted treatment for rheumatoid arthritis in the former Soviet Union.

The importance of the T cell was further reinforced when, in 1987, Dr. Trentham showed that an antibody against T cells, an anti-thymocyte globulin, seemed to alleviate rheumatoid arthritis. Shortly thereafter it was widely agreed that AIDS and rheumatoid arthritis were mutually exclusive diseases.

So that's pretty much where matters stood up to the time of the MIRA study. There was general recognition of the important role played by the T cell, and continued mystery as to what specifically initiates the disease. Prior to the use of antibiotics, most therapies attempted to attack the disease by focusing on this aberrant immune response, provided mainly by T cells. This response can, to some degree, be held in check by certain conventional agents. Scientists were divided on how antibiotics worked, but they were equally in the dark about the mechanism of methotrexate, gold, or other drugs.

MINOCYCLINE AND THE NIH CLINICAL TRIALS

What is the connection between these discoveries and treatment that uses the minocycline form of tetracycline? How did they provide part of the rationale for its further study in the MIRA trials?

Minocycline may help patients with rheumatoid arthritis because it eliminates an infectious agent. Alternatively, arthritis research in animal systems has shown that minocycline affects calcium metabolism or pathways in T cells; and calcium pathways are a critical component of the ways in which T cells activate themselves or function. T cells exposed to minocycline take up too much calcium internally, and then become sick or malfunctional. They seem to quiet down, and the animals go into complete remission or are at least visibly improved by the therapy. This new information favors the possibility that some antibiotic drugs may be beneficial in rheumatoid arthritis because they eliminate these T cell autoimmune responses, and not just because they home in on an infectious agent.

A few years ago, a specific request was issued from NIH headquarters in Bethesda for grant applications that might relate to the infectious theory, and that has been cited as tangible evidence of NIH interest in Dr. Brown's original thesis. Some reasoned the response was slow because many scientists felt at the time that applications would result in little more than a fishing trip. Even at the time of the MIRA trials, most arthritis researchers felt they were still working in the dark. Many of those interested in the disease lacked the aptitude, training, or credentials to explore viruses or related phenomena. Dr. Trentham suggested it would require a scientific consortium to attack the problem, but with the funding difficulties in the present economy it was not a particularly viable prospect.

In the meantime, he predicted, the next generation of research would take its direction from the NIH-sponsored clinical trials of minocycline therapy and other such clinical studies.

REVERSING AN ANCIENT ERROR

What has happened in the field of rheumatology since the direction has finally started to change from the dogma that inflammatory arthritis was a metabolic failure? It was an error that stagnated both scientific inquiry and clinical treatment for a long, long time.

In the preface to a special edition of *Rheumatic Disease Clinics of North America* devoted entirely to "New Directions in Antirheumatic Therapy," Trentham wrote in 1992, "Rheumatology is at a crossroads. It is confronted by a precipitous decline in entrants into the subspecialty. Is the problem solely attributable to the modest economic remuneration inherent to the discipline? I think it is also reflective of past therapeutic patterns of the craft! . . . In the upcoming decades, a shift from dogma to diversity is likely to occur." It went on to list some of the specific articles of past faith that now were being abandoned: "about immune complexes being the cause of autoimmune disease, about the effects of gold, about the role of rheumatoid factor in the etiology of the disease, about the notion that non-steroidal anti-inflammatory drugs (NSAIDs) were all alike, about scleroderma being inevitably fatal. . . ."

Another article he had written for the same publication titled "Rheumatologic therapy for the 1990s: Evolution or Revolution?" notes: ". . . the care of the patient with rheumatic disease in the upcoming decade can be easily perceived as the result of a therapeutic revolution as an orderly succession of new approaches." It was hard to imagine a mainstream medical journal publishing any one of these heresies even as recently as five years earlier. Clearly, the shift was already well under way by the time of the MIRA study.

The drugs that had been considered the standards, even recently, for treating the disease were also being reassessed. A prime mover was a friend and colleague of Trentham at the University of California in San Francisco named Wally Epstein. Using novel epidemiologic methodology, Epstein demonstrated that gold therapy in rheumatoid arthritis actually does nothing to change the outlook for patients with rheumatoid arthritis over the long term. "Our feeling that gold has been so beneficial in the past has been actually incorrect," Trentham said.

Of all the drugs Tom Brown had hated, gold was at the top of the list. If the patient dies of some other cause, then the fact that gold has temporarily masked the symptoms is beneficial. But most patients don't die of some other cause.

Trentham said that Epstein's work represented another change of direction that would be provocative and useful for patients to know about, and in many cases they would learn it from this book before they heard about it from their physicians. "All these people have a little bit of the maverick in them," he said. "Yet Wally is a very well respected professor of medicine and has been in the field for years. He is currently taking some flak for his work, but it was published in one of the most respected journals, *Annals of Internal Medicine,* and he's a first-rate person. It's scientifically legitimate. It's newsworthy. And it has patient-information value. So far he's only dealt with gold; he should go to the others—it's a natural."

One of those other drugs, Trentham knew, was very likely to be methotrexate. He was one of the authors of the lead article when it was first reported in *The New England Journal of Medicine* as an arthritis treatment, and he had had as much experience as anyone in its prescription for connective tissue diseases. Despite the fact that its ancestry as a potent anti-cancer agent still frightened a lot of potential patients, Trentham pointed out that the levels used in arthritis are a small fraction of the dosage for cancer, and the side effects had, over time, proven to be minimal.

Unlike its use in cancer patients, methotrexate doesn't function as a toxin in arthritis, and Trentham didn't consider its Achilles heel to be toxicity. He viewed it as an appropriate drug for most people with severe rheumatoid arthritis, but not one that doctors should prescribe for mild cases. He also acknowledged that because it only works for two or three years there is a finite limitation in its usefulness. When methotrexate is no longer recommended, it isn't because side effects kick in, but because arthritis is an amazingly adaptive disease: there's a rewiring of the circuits, and the disease simply outsmarts it.

Another class of compound, the non-steroidal anti-inflammatory drugs, also entered the arthritis market relatively recently. Buoyed up by claims for safety as a low-risk alternative to prednisone, they soon were being consumed on a daily basis by some nine million arthritics in America alone. It turned out that some of those same people were dying each year from so-called "silent ulcers," and in December of 1988, the Food and Drug Administration estimated the actual NSAID annual mortality rate was as high as 20,000. While a new drug, Cytotec, has apparently solved the ulcer problem and NSAIDs are reportedly much safer now, their debut into the market took a heavy toll.

THE MAKING OF A MAVERICK

In the years since I first met Tom Brown, I have been able to share, sometimes in intimate detail, in two sets of perspectives on what happens to people who have to function in an environment where progress is held hostage by culture. The first was that of Tom's patients, who speak for themselves in the book; the second was the viewpoint of the doctors. Tom was considerably less revealing on this process; he was inclined to view his long struggle more as a phenomenon of nature than as something to be examined closely for the good or the bad in it. He was as clear-eyed as anyone I ever met, but I think he had decided long ago that introspection in adversity could be a handicap, and that it is far less productive to acknowledge personal pain than to be merely relentless. Furthermore, Tom Brown's unique position in his profession was a deliberate choice—and liberating.

Tom hadn't told me much about his own feelings, and I hoped Dr. Trentham might be more accessible. For all his quiet, even self-effacing style, he was clearly a maverick himself, and I suspected his career contained some useful clues on how to break out of the rut of dogma

He said he became involved in his current work out of serendipity. He was trying to make antibodies against joint tissues and discovered that the process re-created rheumatoid arthritis in animals. That was to become his central focus through the years: the possibility that the aberrant immune response is directed to a collagen or cartilage protein.

David Trentham went to college at the University of Tennessee and then stayed there through medical school. He had almost no money, but the school had a fast track program and he was able to become a doctor by the time he was twenty-three, which he acknowledged "is a little unusual." Tennessee had an advanced placement plan in the college and he combined that with the honors program to get through in three years, then did medical school in three as well.

Since 1974 he had been studying rheumatoid arthritis, initially from the viewpoint that collagen is a pivotal auto-antigen in the disease. His research in that area started in Tennessee, but he wanted to look deeper, and that led him to Harvard in 1976. "I came because I felt I could really be in a hotbed of science, that there was a critical mass here." Initially, he joined the staff of the Peter Bent Brigham Hospital, at that time the only free-standing arthritis hospital in the country. There was a lot of science going on there as well, and he continued his research at Brigham for the next ten years.

Along the way, he became interested in learning—assuming the crucial influence in rheumatoid arthritis was collagen activity—the mechanism to which it was subservient. That led him into the field of T cells and involvement in a number of therapeutic trials, which, in turn, brought him to his present interest in minocycline. Trentham's work with T cells in rheumatoid arthritis pre-dated T cell theory in AIDS research by several years. Largely based on the work Paulus had done with thoracic duct drainage and Boxel's observations, it began in 1976 and 1977.

Trentham got a fair share of the right kind of encouragement. Larry Shulman at the NIH and Claude Bennett, chief of medicine at the University of Alabama, supplied the link between antibiotic therapy and rheumatoid arthritis. Back in the '60s and early '70s, when he was very active as an investigator, Bennett had worked on mycoplasma and rheumatoid arthritis. Bennett and Shulman were both extremely interested in antibiotics and prodded Trentham to take a closer look in that direction.

For all the similarities in their approach to the disease, Trentham was largely unaware of Thomas McPherson Brown. Back in 1975, Trentham's knowledge of Brown's work was at best peripheral, limited almost entirely to disparaging remarks by other colleagues. "The fact is, I really felt he must have been some kind of a crazy, a charlatan, and what he was doing at that point was of no interest to me whatsoever."

Shulman and Bennett urged him to submit a grant application to the NIH. They felt the whole field needed further inquiry. They informed Trentham of Larry Golub, a dental researcher at SUNY in Stony Brook, whose research proved that minocycline was a calcium chelator (a binding agent that suppresses chemical activity), which, in tests, suppressed some deleterious enzyme release in collagenates. Collagenase is known to the laity as a meat tenderizer, and it is probable that this tendency for breaking down tissue is, in part, responsible for the destruction of the joints in rheumatoid arthritis patients.

Trentham reasoned that Golub's findings helped to explain scattered anecdotal claims that minocycline was useful in treating rheumatoid arthritis. He sought out a few of the authors of these reports, like Lee Bartholomew, who at that time was at the medical college at Albany and by the time of the MIRA trials was semiretired in upstate New York. Bartholomew also had studied mycoplasma in rheumatoid arthritis and published a paper in about 1965 on isolating it from synovial fluid. When he tried again he couldn't reproduce his results, however, and he began to have doubts, principally that his first success might have actually been a contaminant. But Bartholomew still felt there was something there, and he, too, encouraged Trentham to take a further look into the area.

Up to then, Trentham had been unwilling to explore the infectious theory in animals because he thought the model would be so distant from humans that the information would not be extrapolatable, and he also felt he lacked the training or background to pursue infectious agents himself. But in combination, the new incentives proved irresistible. He was excited

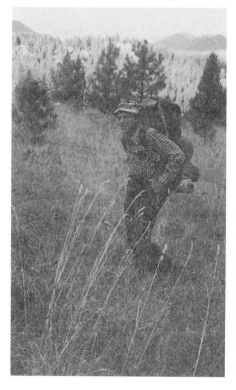

Clarence Kassens of Colville, Wash., will be eighty on his next birthday. He suffered from rheumatoid arthritis for twenty years, but after an acute flareup he heard of antibiotic therapy in 1992.

Since then, I have felt very good—literally have not even had a cold or a sniffle. I am exercising regularly and my strength and endurance are improving. The permanent damage to my right hip socket is still there, so I no longer do any jogging. However, I am still bicycling and hiking with a moderate pack. I feel very fortunate in being able to get started on the right treatment. If it had not been for this, by now I would probably be crippled or bedridden.

about the possibility that collagen reactivity appeared to play an important role in the disease; he had reason to believe that minocycline might work in a way that hadn't been explored before, and he had been interested in T cells for over a decade. A study of animal models of rheumatoid arthritis produced by collagen, determining whether minocycline really produced the benefits reported in the anecdotes, could have great predictive value for human treatment. Along the way, he would focus on whether minocycline also influenced T cells in the same model. In 1968 he was awarded a grant from the NIH for three years.

It did everything he had hoped for. He showed that tetracyclines are effective in animals, just as Tom Brown had demonstrated when he had used the same antibiotics to cure Tomoka, the gorilla at the National Zoo. He also identified the changes in calcium metabolism that might explain the event.

REMEMBER THE ALAMO

David Trentham was forty-seven years old when the code was broken on the double-blind clinical trials of minocycline in 1993. The MIRA study was scheduled as the lead presentation at that year's scientific meeting of the American College of Rheumatology, and when the moment came the San Antonio auditorium was filled to its 5,000-seat capacity. Floating high in the void above the darkened stage, massive televised images of the speakers were projected onto three enormous screens, and impeccable acoustics carried their voices with face-to-face clarity into every corner of the hall. With the president of the ACR serving as emcee, the statistician from Detroit, Barbara Tilley, the only non-medical doctor on the study team and an unlikely Moses, took her place in the circle of light.

Her presentation was limited to only a few minutes, but for those in the audience who had been waiting for this moment for years before the MIRA trials were conceived, the results (see "Let's Start with the Proof") were electrifying. As questioners lined up in long queues behind two microphones in the aisles, the name of Dr. Thomas McPherson Brown was invoked repeatedly. The emcee, no doubt in the spirit of fairness and on a tight schedule, began responding to such mentions of the ACR's old nemesis by cutting in and requesting the speaker to state his question.

By the third or fourth time this happened, one of the participants who knew I had been Tom Brown's co-author grinned at me from across the aisle and rolled his eyes in amusement.

It would be another fifteen months before the MIRA study would at last appear in print.

Is It Safe?

Does the question sound familiar?

Millions of moviegoers remember it as the sinister, oft-repeated query by the fugitive Nazi physician played by Laurence Olivier in *Marathon Man*. Every time the White Angel asks Dustin Hoffman's young student, "Is it safe?" none of us thinks for a minute that it is out of any concern for the well-being of his intended victim. Quite the contrary—the evil doctor, up from the jungles of Paraguay to cash in his trove of stolen diamonds, hardly expects the Hoffman character to live through dinner.

This same question illuminates one of those areas of medicine in which life frequently imitates art. In evaluating risk versus benefit, physicians always weigh the perils to themselves as well as to the patient, and if there is a conflict, the patient's interests usually will come in second. Regardless of how many times a standard therapy has been proven worthless or even downright dangerous, it's still a lot safer *for the doctor* than prescribing any modality that has not yet gained acceptance in a particular application. It equally doesn't matter how many times a therapy may have been applied successfully in an off-label use, or even if it has demonstrated the potential for saving the patient's life. Their own professional security is the sole reason that some of the same doctors who consider tetracycline safe enough to prescribe for millions of adolescents with nothing more serious than pimples will unblushingly question its safety in the treatment of a disease that can cripple or kill.

Dr. Thomas McPherson Brown was an exception. Over the course of his long career he prescribed the off-label use of antibiotics to some 10,000 patients with connective tissue disease. He knew as well as everyone else in medicine that tetracyclines are famous for their benign profile, and he had "not seen any toxic effects in forty years in anybody." Nor did one of those many patients ever complain of a single instance of malpractice or misfeasance. Indeed, dermatologist Alan R. Cantwell, Jr., describes antibiotic therapy as "far safer than steroids, aspirin, non-steroidal anti-inflammatory agents, gold, and methotrexate."

Tetracyclines, in common with any other medicine, can sometimes have side effects, but beyond sun sensitivity during the course of therapy and occasional vaginal yeast infections in women (easily corrected with nothing more drastic than a small helping of yogurt), adverse responses are rare and few. The antibiotic can cause transient dizziness and stomach queasiness, and occasional discoloration of the skin and, in young children, of the teeth. More serious reactions, such as hypersensitivity syndrome reaction, serum sickness, and what has been described as a drug-induced form of lupus, occur with such infrequency that they collectively amount to a tiny fraction of one percent of the number of the far more deadly complaints associated with non-steroidal anti-inflammatories (NSAIDs) alone. There are contraindications for the use of any medicine, but most practitioners, like Cantwell, "have never heard of anyone becoming seriously ill with tetracycline, or even minocycline."

The claim that tetracyclines are safer than any of the other therapies is more than a figure of speech. Conventional treat-

ments for rheumatoid arthritis can be more devastating than
the affliction they purport to treat. Just a few weeks after publication of *The Road Back*, *Newsweek* ran a cover story on the
finding by the Food and Drug Administration that NSAIDs
were killing up to 20,000 Americans a year. That was considerably more people than the number then believed to die annu-
ally from arthritis, and was equal to the mortality estimates for
the far rarer scleroderma. NSAIDs were reformulated that
same year and the losses were cut by an estimated 85 percent,
but that "more acceptable" level still leaves a death rate equal
to the crash of a fully loaded jumbo jet once every month.

For another comparison, consider Pat Ganger's experience
with d-penicillamine. Although her initial response to the drug
was that in the first year it seemed to help with the soreness and
produced a slight loosening of the skin, those benefits proved
transitory. It was well established that penicillamine can cause
problems with blood cell production in the bone marrow, but
with the continued hardening of her skin that risk became
impossible to monitor. Moreover, up to the time she stopped
treatment after five years of ineffectual therapy, not a single
placebo-controlled, double-blind clinical study of this drug had
ever been conducted to determine whether it was worth doing
in the first place. When such trials finally were completed on
penicillamine in scleroderma some eight years after Pat had
quit, they simply proved what she and many others knew
already: the drug did virtually nothing to halt the long-term
progress of the disease.

Let's look at methotrexate, which was initially developed to
battle cancer. The 1987 study by Tugwell, Bennett, and Gent
reported nausea, vomiting, anorexia, diarrhea, stomatitis,
leukopenia, anemia, thrombocytopenia, toxicity of the liver, kidneys, or lungs, possible malignancy, reduced sperm production,
excessive development of male breasts, fever, localized osteoporosis, and leukocytonbastic vasculitis.

This chapter opened with a memory test, so let's close it the
same way. How many of us can recall thalidomide? Even if you
weren't around when this sedative/hypnotic first appeared on

the scene a generation ago, you probably recognize the name as a paradigm for the unthinkable. Although thalidomide was never officially approved by the FDA, large amounts of the drug were brought into this country for personal use by visitors returning from the United Kingdom, where it was available in pharmacies by prescription. Some of those travelers, or their friends in America with whom they shared this forbidden apple, were women, and some of those women were pregnant.

But was it safe?

Britons found out the answer before we did, because they started using thalidomide sooner. At first the horrific results were kept quiet, but even if they had been disclosed immediately it wouldn't have made that much difference. By the time the public realized they had bitten into a worm, it was too late. Up to 12,000 expectant mothers on both sides of the Atlantic who had taken the drug to help them get to sleep, including some who had used it only once or twice, gave birth to malformed babies, some without eyes or ears, many with limbs that were severely truncated or missing entirely. Uncounted thousands more elected to end their pregnancies, some on the knowledge that the fetus was malformed, and some simply on the risk that it might be. It was one of the most tragic mass poisonings in the history of medicine.

Even if the general public doesn't have a terrific collective memory, we can be sure the pharmaceutical industry hasn't forgotten its experience with thalidomide any more than Union Carbide is likely to forget Bhopal or Exxon will forget the *Valdez* disaster. However, it has been observed that history, like character, is not determined by triumphs or calamities alone, but by what happens next. And what is happening next with the admirably resilient industry that brought us thalidomide the first time? They're bringing it back.

As of this writing, volunteers are being sought through notices in hospitals, medical journals, and letters, and on the Internet to participate in a new twelve-week therapeutic study of this drug in the United States. "All women of child-bearing age must have a negative pregnancy test at the screening and must practice effective contraception for at least one month prior to study entry," the call specifies, "with at least two forms of birth control (an oral or implanted contraceptive and a barrier method) while part of the study. During the study all women in this age group will receive biweekly pregnancy tests."

These days the drug isn't being tested for how well it helps women get to sleep, but on whether it does anything useful for scleroderma. Similar tests are under consideration for rheumatoid arthritis.

"Why on earth would anyone test a drug on our disease when it is already known to have such terrible side effects?" one scleroderma patient asked when she heard about the thalidomide study. "Do they think most of us are too young to remember? Or have they decided that as a group, because we're probably going to die anyway, we represent a different level of risk?"

_____

CHAPTER 34.

Tailoring the Therapy

There is a temptation in medicine, as elsewhere in life, to believe that if something is found to be good for us, more of it is even better. Sometimes that's true, and sometimes it's not. The early history of anti-inflammatories and antibiotics, for two examples, saw prescriptions written for many times the dosage levels that subsequently proved effective on the disease or even safe for the patient. More recent experience has seen the opposite.

Prednisone, which responsible physicians today dole out in 5- or 10-milligram tablets to help manage the discomfort or pain of inflammation, was initially prescribed in doses as much as 80 or 100 times higher—and sometimes still is. By the time a patient with a connective tissue disease is no longer able to tolerate the therapy, which can happen very soon at those high levels, the prognosis is likely to be complicated by cataracts, weak, unhealthy "cortisone skin," and kidney failure. When susceptibility to any of these same problems is also a characteristic of the disease, such as skin anomalies or renal collapse in the case of scleroderma, the problem is compounded. Moreover, because the treatment of external effects can merely mask the disease without doing anything for its cause, the original problem has usually gotten far worse by the time the suppressed symptoms suddenly return with a vengeance. A prolonged heavy hand can also burn out the body's ability to manufacture anti-inflammatories on its own, so the unnatural dependency becomes permanent.

For some of the same reasons, too much of an antibiotic can create more problems than it cures. But conversely, as has been demonstrated in recent experience with Lyme disease, so can *under*prescribing either the dosage level or the duration of therapy. Choosing the right drug is only part of the solution. Also important is the development of an appropriate protocol for its administration.

The way most medical protocols are established is by trial and error, by varying the parameters and observing the results, keeping track of what works and what doesn't. Regardless of what it says on the bottle, many doctors adjust dosage levels, frequencies, and even routes of administration to the needs and responses of the patient, with the ultimate goal of reducing the amount as quickly as possible and as far as possible while still controlling the disease. But in the short term the adjustment can go up or down.

In 1988, Carol Lange experienced a severe flare of rheumatoid arthritis, a disease that her doctor, Thomas McPherson Brown, had been controlling with antibiotics for the previous twenty-four years. Dr. Brown knew that flareups, in common with fast-moving or severe diseases as well as all forms of scleroderma, require aggressive intervention. As usual, he started her off with 300 milligrams of clindamycin administered intravenously the first day, then 600 the second, and 900 every day for the balance of the week, along with her regular course of oral minocycline, and the flareup slowly receded. (At a recent conference of physicians experienced in antibiotic therapy for scleroderma and other connective tissue diseases, there was a consensus that this combination approach was the most effective in dealing with such extremes.) But Dr. Brown died a short time later, and Carol had to find another doctor.

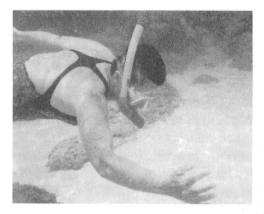

Carol Lange, artist, teacher, administrator, Glasboro, N.J. Now fifty-eight, she was diagnosed with severe RA while still in high school.

Eight years later, early in the winter of 1964, my right knee, left hand, and shoulder dramatically flared and in three weeks I lost the use of my left arm. The local doctor tried anti-malarial and anti-inflammatory drugs, but by March I was told I probably had six months before I would need a wheelchair, then downhill from there to total care. I was twenty-four years old. Thank God my rheumatologist referred me to the Dean of Medicine at George Washington University Medical School, Dr. Thomas McPherson Brown.

After an examination, history, and blood tests, Dr. Brown said, "If you stick with my treatment, I promise you'll get back the use of your arm. Meanwhile, you worry about your sculpture and I'll worry about your arthritis." That was our "deal" for the next twenty-five years. Today, despite an occasional flare, I am in control of my disease, lead a useful, productive life, and have full use of all my joints.

This time the physician was Albert Dawkins, a rheumatologist in nearby Maryland who had worked with Brown at George Washington University Medical School, first as a protégé and then as a colleague, and had developed a considerable body of his own experience in treating hundreds of arthritis patients with antibiotic therapy. He handled Carol's next flareup with the same drug and at the same dosage level as were used by Brown, but with her assent, and based on his success with other patients he doubled the frequency to twice a day and extended it two days longer. He also combined the antibiotic therapy with an NSAID and an antihistamine, both administered orally. The approach worked so well that whenever Carol had a flareup over the following years, she and Dawkins could predict its course with nearly clockwork accuracy. At the fifth day, following her Herxheimer reaction, they would see a remarkable reduction in her pain and related disease activity, and she would walk out of the hospital completely reversed, pain-free and with no disabilities at the end of the treatment.

Both Dr. Dawkins and Carol understood that the Herxheimer was a temporary, drug-dose-induced flareup and not a toxic reaction to the drug. Carol had agreed to ride out the discomfort in order to achieve a long-term benefit from the elevated dosage. Among other things, finding the right combination comes down to the doctor's experience with the therapy and the patient's history and levels of tolerance.

As of this writing, most physicians have never prescribed minocycline for connective tissue disease, which means that some will now be looking for guidelines to that application. But this is not a case where one size fits all: not everyone is the same age, weight, height, race, or gender, they don't share a common immune system, and they don't have identical medical histories. Regardless of what guidelines a doctor follows for any drug, it is commonplace to adjust the parameters of dosage, frequency, term, and sometimes combinations with other medicines to the needs of each patient. For obvious reasons, such variations are not permissible in a controlled study, but in their clinical practices rheumatologists do it all the time with prednisone, Naprosyn, methotrexate, plaquenil, penicillamine, gold salts, and all the other drugs they prescribe for arthritis and every other connective tissue disease.

Less commonplace in medicine, however, is the use of antibiotics over a prolonged period of time. Although most rheumatologists are comfortable offering any of the above nostrums for as long as the patient can tolerate them before losing liver or kidney function or going blind, most schedules for the use of antibiotics in the treatment of infectious disease are no longer than a week or ten days. There's a good reason for this restraint in the use of antibiotics in general: ten days is usually long enough to do the job, and overusing them can encourage the development of resistant strains of the bugs they were designed to kill.

But as we have already seen, minocycline is not like most other antibiotics. Tom Brown learned from his earliest experience with the elusive L-forms that they were capable of such astonishing tenacity, it was sometimes necessary to keep up the antibiotic pressure for months and even years. To gain any lasting, measurable benefits with as brief a regimen as ten days is nearly impossible.

During periods when the patients were hospitalized for intensive therapy, Dr. Brown concentrated the treatment for maximum impact, and for the same reasons Dr. Dawkins took an even more aggressive approach at such times. But for the maintenance programs by which this therapy was administered the rest of the time, most other experienced doctors, including Dawkins, followed Brown's technique of spacing the doses in response to the needs of the patient. At one point Carol Lange was on a schedule of five days of medication followed by two days off, and at other times she was on every other day, every third day, or two on and one off; the most common schedule was three times a week, with nothing on Saturdays and Sundays.

The principle behind this irregular schedule was based on the fact that tetracycline will stay in the body for forty-eight hours or more after oral administration. The spacing allowed the body to rest between doses without losing the cumulative impact of the antibiotic, which is held in low-metabolizing tissues such as bones and cartilage where it can still be drawn into the system, albeit at lower levels, even on days when no drug is given. The Road Back Foundation recently developed a graph showing the relationship between the peaking of antibiotic activity and the subsequent peaking of antigenic activity with the use of minocycline. Daily doses create a relatively steady condition in which the minocycline might be expected to initiate a hypersensitivity reaction, while alternating doses avoids the overlapping effect and can sometimes, although not always, allow the hypersensitivity reaction to remit. Likewise, too much antibiotic at any one time can trigger a similar problem that is often relieved by nothing more complex than an adjustment in the dose.

Dr. Brown's longtime laboratory director, Harold Clark, says two other advantages of the pulse method are that the off days give the body tissues a respite from the oxidation associated with the use of antibiotics, as well as providing an interim for restoration of normal protein synthesis in the cells. Mycoplasmas are relatively lethargic reproducers, so any such small hiatus is unlikely to encourage a breeding spree.

One other factor to consider in the use of any drug, particularly antibiotics, is the huge differences in effectiveness that can sometimes exist between the original branded product and its generic counterpart. The FDA requires that any generic form must have a bioequivalence within twenty percent of the drug it copies, which means that two generic versions of the same drug can vary from each other by as much as forty percent in effectiveness. This can be especially problematical in the case of minocycline, which can be chemically equivalent under the law but miss the mark altogether in terms of clinical benefits with diseases as complex as inflammatory arthritis, lupus, or scleroderma. In RA, very often the only difference between a response and a non-response to minocycline is whether the prescription is filled with the original Lederle formulation, branded as Minocin, or a generic dud.

CHAPTER 35

In Defense of Heresy

There's an old story about a policeman who encounters a drunk at around midnight, down on his hands and knees searching the sidewalk under a streetlamp. When questioned, the drunk says he's looking for a silver dollar he dropped an hour earlier at the other end of the block. "So what are you doing down here?" the officer asks. "Why aren't you looking where you lost it?"

"Use your head, man," the searcher replies, squinting into the void beyond the ring of the streetlamp. "It's as black as the pit out there. What chance would I have of finding it in the dark?"

You can see that same joke repeated every day on every well-lighted street corner in medicine. Searchers by the thousands scour the same old territory for as long as the light lasts, in some rare cases just to prove the ground is fallow, but far more often for no better reason than the certainty that even when they come up empty-handed they still get paid for looking.

And what about the far fewer researchers who are actually willing to work in the dark where answers await discovery, the true scientists who are led by a hunch or happenstance to challenge a tradition or consensus that is always heavily defended by politics and myth? They can be assured of a very hard road: shunning or outright attacks by colleagues who frequently are also their rivals, little or no grant support, restricted access or no access to peer-reviewed media, loss of reputation, frequently loss of income, and sometimes loss of employment.

When the producer of "20/20" asked Tom Brown why he had written a book for the general public that challenged the conventional view of connective tissue disease after four decades of nearly constant attack by the medical establishment for those very same heresies, he answered with a tired smile, "Because I've finally outlived the sons of bitches." But of course, he had not. The real reason Tom wrote the book was because he knew he was dying. If there was any doubt of the outcome, by the time the segment aired it was abundantly apparent the sons of bitches were going to outlive the pioneer. They usually do.

In 1984, Dr. Barry Marshall was serving out his residency at a hospital in Perth, Australia. At about the same age as Tom Brown and Albert Sabin had been when they began their careers at the Rockefeller Institute some half-century earlier, he too made a discovery that one day would revolutionize medicine. Suspecting that bacteria, not stress, were the cause of stomach ulcers, he and a colleague had taken samples from the stomachs of ulcer patients and were trying to culture something in a Petri dish. The standard incubation time is forty-eight hours, and like Tom Brown with mycoplasma, they had come up empty in their first several attempts to isolate a potential culprit. By chance, however, over the Easter holidays one batch was left in its dish for more than twice the normal length of time, and they returned to find a colony of corkscrew-like *Helicobacter pylori* swarming under the microscope. Repeating the technique, the same suspect appeared in cultures from other ulcer patients.

The obvious next step in Koch's postulate would be to use the bacteria to induce this disease in an animal model, as Sabin had induced arthritis with his second mouse, but those attempts proved just as unproductive as their earlier tries at culturing the bug. In frustration, young Dr. Marshall decided, perhaps rashly, to try the experiment on a human subject, swilling down a microbial cocktail that he later described as tasting like swamp water. A week later he awoke in the middle of the night with severe stomach cramps, and a few days after that an endoscopic examination with a tiny TV camera revealed a gastric inflammation of the type often associated with ulcers.

Armed with these revolutionary results, Marshall hit the medical convention trail to rouse the sleeping populace—and of course his colleagues responded to the wake-up call with nudges, winks, and snickers. Who was this bothersome upstart? He came from a hospital hardly anyone had ever heard of, was still a resident, hardly even a clinician and certainly not a researcher. Everybody knew that ulcers were caused by acid triggered by stress (one way of blaming the patient, as stress is usually seen as a function of lifestyle.) There had been a long-standing myth in medicine that the environment of the stomach was too hostile to support any life forms, and many doctors still adhered to that fiction even though it had been disproven before Barry Marshall ever appeared on their horizon.

Perhaps even more to the point, there was already an absolutely wonderful treatment, Tagamet, an acid-blocker approved by the FDA less than a decade earlier that had cut ulcer surgery by a third in its first year on the market and that by 1984 had become the best-selling drug on earth. From a strictly business point of view, the real magic of acid blockers was that no matter how many times they "cured" the disease, the ulcers usually came back. No investor in his right mind would want to kill the goose that lays that kind of golden annuity, and neither, apparently, would the typical gastroenterologist for whom ulcers produced a quarter of all annual income.

The more resistance he met, the more determined Dr. Marshall became. He concocted a number of different therapies aimed at knocking out both the painful symptoms and the *H. pylori,* which he remained convinced was their real cause. He got a 70 percent remission rate with a combination of Pepto-Bismol and the antibiotic metronidazole, and when someone else added tetracycline to the mix the effectiveness rose another 15 points to 85 percent of all stomach ulcers treated, a number that may represent 100 percent of those with a bacterial etiology.

Unlike Tom Brown, he responded to the indifference or criticism of his colleagues by turning up the volume, often angrily scolding them at medical conventions about their obligation as healers to eradicate ulcers at their source, an exercise that increased his visibility in about the same degree as it reduced his peer popularity. But eventually his efforts began to attract a different constituency, and a far larger audience. After he published a paper in the British medical journal *The Lancet*, the story of his work was picked up in America by *The National Enquirer*, then the *Cincinnati Enquirer*, and eventually the *Wall Street Journal*. For many, his saga became a model of everything that was wrong with how the establishment responded to innovation, how the ethics of medicine had been pre-empted by the venality of big business, and how the little guy, whether a renegade genius or a helpless patient, always gets it in the neck. It was one of the best conspiracy stories since the assassination of John F. Kennedy, only this time the victim was still alive and it looked as if he finally had a chance of winning.

A decade and a half after that breakthrough in Perth, how has this process played itself out: how is Dr. Marshall viewed in the medical establishment, and how much of a difference have discovering the cause of stomach ulcers and offering an effective cure made in the way the disease is now treated?

Today it is almost universally accepted that 85 percent of all ulcers in the digestive system are caused by the bacteria he identified in 1984, and numerous clinical trials have shown that antibiotic therapy can cure them up to 100 percent of the time. Meanwhile, *H. pylori* have also been implicated in stomach cancer, which, in parts of the world such as Italy and Peru where the bacteria are more ubiquitous, can be a leading cause of death. In America, the NIH has officially declared that ulcer patients with *H. pylori* should have the bacteria eradicated.

Procter & Gamble, which had acquired Pepto-Bismol, began supporting Dr. Marshall when they recognized that his work with bismuth against *H. pylori* might represent an opportunity to carve out a larger share in their new pharmaceutical marketplace, and under the company's powerful aegis the young renegade from Perth moved into a new position at the University of Virginia Medical School. Even though his work met with often blistering criticism, ridicule, and even personal attacks at every step of the way, almost all of his original critics have swung full circle, some gracefully and some grudgingly, in support of the infectious theory and antibiotic therapy. In 1995 he was honored with the prestigious Lasker Award for his work on ulcers, and three years later many people still consider him a prime candidate for the Nobel Prize in medicine.

All of which might appear to be the happiest possible ending to these two stories, both of a truly deserving innovator and of the scourge that he has devoted his career to eradicating.

But so far, that would be a false conclusion. Despite all the well-publicized evidence of its efficacy, safety, and cost-effectiveness, the number of ulcer cases actually treated by antibiotic therapy had risen only sluggishly, from zero in 1984 to a mere 16 percent in 1995, a share described by *Fortune* magazine as "amazingly few." Dr. Marshall's office at the medical school still receives panicked telephone calls from patients who are facing painful, expensive, and life-threatening surgery for a condition that the world now knows can be treated better medically, and at far less cost or risk. If the young Australian doctor ever does make it down the aisle at Oslo, it is a certainty that those plaintive calls for help will be ringing louder in his mind than anything he is likely to be hearing at the same time from his colleagues, whether their praise, their familiar but subdued snickers, or the gnashing of old teeth.

In his classic work, *The Structure of Scientific Revolutions*, the late MIT professor Thomas S. Kuhn sees the process outlined above—and indeed, the process described in this brief book—as being not just occasional to such change, but inevitable. "Normal science," he writes, "often suppresses fun-

Dona Morris, sixty-one, is a police clerk in De Queen, Ark. She developed symptoms of systemic scleroderma in 1989 and was diagnosed in April 1990.

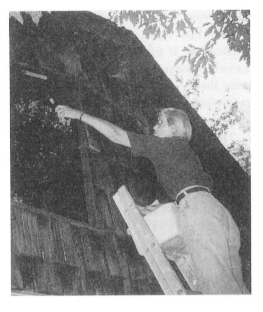

Things moved fast; in a year I had severe joint pains, problems swallowing and breathing, extreme fatigue, contractures of the fingers, ulcerated joints, and hardening or tightening of the skin all over my body. I saw a series of rheumatologists, but none of them could offer a thing that helped. I finally found a doctor who put me on antibiotic therapy in January 1991.

I was pretty far along when they started me on IVs, and they had to push so hard to get the needle through my skin, there was a risk of blowing the vein. But it began to work almost from the start. The redness and soreness left my hands, the skin softened, and the ulcers healed on my knuckles. The lung and throat problems got better, along with my range of motion. The nurses giving the treatment were amazed at the difference in my condition.

Today, all I have left of this disease are contractures in one hand and some thickened tissue on part of one leg. I can do things at work, around the house, and in the garden that I never expected to do again. My life has been given back to me.

damental novelties because they are necessarily subversive of its basic commitments." He describes the major turning points in the careers of Copernicus, Newton, Lavoisier, and Einstein, among many others, as dramas in which the transforming event results not just from insight or serendipity but from the resolution of the often bitter contest between personalities, between the cultures of the status quo and the revolutionary, between deeply entrenched and heavily defended traditions that no longer work and radical changes that do, between the present and the future: ". . . a new theory, however special its range of application, is seldom or never just an increment of what is already known. Its assimilation requires the reconstruction of prior theory and the re-evaluation of prior fact, an intrinsically revolutionary process that is seldom completed by a single man and never overnight."

That contest can be vastly more complex when the science is in medicine, and the outcome of a medical revolution frequently depends far more on the strength of its champions than on the power of its truth.

Consider the case of Virginia Wuerthele-Caspe, M.D. (later and better known as Virginia Livingston-Wheeler), the lead author some years back, along with Eva Brodkin, M.D., and Camille Mermod, M.D., of a preliminary clinical report titled *Etiology of Scleroderma*. The study was based on the probable bacterial cause of scleroderma and its treatment with antibacterial agents.

"On the assumption that the organism is a mycobacterium as in leprosy and tuberculosis," she wrote, "the senior author reasoned that it should be found in nasal ulcers, subcutaneous tissue, and sputum when there is pulmonary involvement. Accordingly material was prepared from the sputum of a proved case of scleroderma. When the slides were stained by the Ziehl-Neelson method, numerous short, thick, acid-fast rods appeared." A cooperating team of investigators was formed to study the organism's pathology in six patients, all but one of whom were women.

The conclusions of the study, potentially at least, were revolutionary in the true sense of the word. "An acid-fast bacillus [was] found in five cases of scleroderma examined bacteriologically. The organism [was] found in the sputum, blood, nasal and subcutaneous tissue smears, and has been grown in pure culture from the blood. All patients treated with promin (which destroys or inhibits mycobacteria) have shown definite, responsive changes. The organism . . . may be a newly recognized member of the family of mycobacteria."

So whatever happened to these four muses, the first researchers to name mycoplasmas as the prime suspect in the disease of scleroderma and the first to point directly to antibiotics as a therapy that works?

In case you missed it, all three authors of the study are women, as is the researcher in charge of the lab work, a questionable advantage in medicine even in today's enlightened environment. And what they are reporting, in its context, is revolutionary, which means they are also heretics.

Because the authors were deprived of virtually all the power required for effective advocacy, although their brilliant, prescient study was knocking at the door to a cure of this disease, it failed to meet the acid test of What Happened Next. It was published, not in *JAMA* or *The Lancet* or *Arthritis and Rheumatism*, but in *The Journal of the Medical Society of New Jersey*. And it appeared in print long before the term "glass ceiling" had been coined and before *PC* meant either politically correct or personal computer, a half-century ago, in the summer of 1947. And of course it was universally ignored.

Now, over a million scleroderma patients later, another study has been completed, this one pointing more directly to a cure for the disease; the fact that you are now reading this book means that the scientific report of The Road Back Foundation's scleroderma study at Harvard Medical School has already been presented in a peer-reviewed medical forum. This time the revolutionary concept may have some advantage in its aegis, but it is revolutionary nonetheless and will hardly be exempted from the protracted and surely rancorous defense of the truths that it will eventually displace.

On May 8, 1998, at the Sixth Biennial Meeting of the International Society for Rheumatic Therapy in Boston—in the same forum and on the same day that David Trentham presented the results of the Harvard Medical School study of minocycline in scleroderma—a kind of requiem was offered for the long, mean war against the use of that drug in rheumatoid arthritis. Sheldon Cooper, M.D., of the University of Vermont Medical School presented a paper titled

"Minocycline for RA: The Controversy is Gone." Dr. Cooper, who ran one of the six treatment centers in the MIRA study and who is emerging as a key figure in the ascent of antibiotic therapy, was obviously deliberate in his choice of such an optimistic title, and it wasn't hard to imagine the reaction it would engender among the majority of his profession, who remain far more faithful to ancient folly. But if the title was more prophetic than factual, it acknowledged that a foot is now firmly wedged in a door that had been nailed shut for decades, and promised that someday soon there would be enough such feet to kick it down.

Similarly, the purpose of this book is to broaden the forum in which the new truths are weighed against the old by inviting in the thousands of patients for whom this therapy can mean the difference between improvement or remission and crippling pain, and sometimes between life and death. For doctors or patients, the experience and insights of others who have traveled a similar road can illuminate personal choices that ease the journey.

At the bottom line, all patients are consumers, whatever the name of their disease, and they deserve not just to participate but to be in charge of the process by which they select the most appropriate therapy and hire the best physician to provide it.

They no longer have to take no for an answer.

The Studies

(Courtesy Pat Ganger and The Road Back Foundation)

RA TRIALS

Minocycline Treatment for Rheumatoid Arthritis: An Open Dose Finding Study, FC Breedveld, BAC Dijkmans, H Mattie, *J Rheum*, 1990, 17:1, 43-46

Treatment of Resistant Rheumatoid Arthritis with Minocycline: An Open Study, P. Langevitz, I Bank, D Zemer, M Book, M Pras, *J Rheum*, 1992; 19:10, 1502-1504.

Antibiotics as Disease Modifiers in Arthritis, M Kloppenburg, AMM Miltenburg, BAC Dijkmans, *Clin Exper Rheum II*, 1993 (Suppl. 8): S113-S115.

Minocycline in Active Rheumatoid Arthritis: A Double-Blind, Placebo-Controlled Study, M Kloppenburg, FC Breedveld, JPh Terwiel, C Mallee, BAC Dijkmans, H Mattie, *Arth & Rheum*, 1994; 37:5, 629-636.

Minocycline in Rheumatoid Arthritis: A 48-Week, Double-Blind, Placebo-Controlled Trial, BC Tilley, GS Alarcon, SP Heyse, DE Trentham, R Neuner, DA Kaplan, DO Clegg, JCC Leisen, L Buckley, SM Cooper, H Duncan, SR Pillemer, M Tuttleman, SE Fowler, *Ann Int Med*, Jan. 15, 1995, 122:2, 81-89.

Minocycline Treatment of Rheumatoid Arthritis (editorial), HE Paulus, *Ann Int Med*, Jan. 15, 1995, 122:2, 147-148.

Minocycline in the Treatment of Rheumatoid Arthritis: Relationship of Serum Concentrations to Efficacy, M Kloppenburg, H Mattie, N Douwes, BAC Dijkmans, FC Breedveld, *J Rheum*, 1995; 22:4, 611-616.

Successful Treatment of Early Rheumatoid Arthritis (RA) with Minocycline: Results of a Double-Blind Trial, J O'Dell, C Haire, N Erickson, W Palmer, M Churchill, W Drymalski, K Blakely, S Wees, J Eckhoff, D Doud, A Weaver, F Dietz, R Olson, L Klassen, G Moore, *Arth & Rheum*, 1995, 40:5, 842-848.

Minocycline in Rheumatoid Arthritis (editorial), FC Breedveld, *Arth & Rheum*, 1995, 40:5, 794-796.

Minocycline in Rheumatoid Arthritis, P Langevitz, A Livneh, I Bank, M Pras, *Isr J Med Sci*, 1996; 32: 327-330.

Meaningful Improvement Criteria Sets in a Rheumatoid Arthritis Clinical Trial, SR Pillemer, SE Fowler, BC Tilley, GS Alarcon, SP Heyse, DE Trentham, R Neuner, DO Clegg, JC Liesen, SM Cooper, H Duncan, M Tuttleman, *Arth & Rheum*, 1997; 40:3, 419-425.

Minocycline Therapy for Early Rheumatoid Arthritis (RA): Continued Efficacy at Three Years, J O'Dell, C Hair, N Erickson, W Palmer, M Churchill, W Drymalski, K Blakely, S Wees, J Eckhoff, D Doud, A Weaver, F Dietz, R Olson, L Klassen, G Moore (abstract), *Arth & Rheum*, Nov 1997.

OTHER RA STUDIES

Possible Role of *Mycoplasma Fermentans* in Pathogenesis of Rheumatoid Arthritis, MH Williams, J Bristoff, IM Roitt, *Lancet*, Aug. 8, 1970, 277-280.

An 8-Year Study on Mycoplasma in Rheumatoid Arthritis, E Jansson, P Makisara, K Vainio, U Vainio, O Snellman, Sirkka Tuuri, *Ann Rheum Dis*, 1971, 30:506-508.

Mycoplasmas and Bacteria in Synovial Fluid from Patients with Arthritis, PA Mardh, FJ Nilsson, A Bielle, *Ann Rheum Dis*, 1973, 32; 319-325.

Progress in Understanding of Inducible Models of Chronic Arthritis, FC Breedveld, DE Trentham, *Rheum Dis Clin of N Am*, 1987; 13:3, 531-544.

The Microbial Causes of Rheumatoid Arthritis, D Ford, *J Rheum*, 1991; 18:10, 1441-1442.

Mycoplasmas and Arthritis, K Hakkarainen, et al, *Ann Rheum Dis*, 1992; 51: 1170-1172.

The Microbial Cause of Rheumatoid Arthritis: Time to Dump Koch's Postulates P Tan, M Skinner, *J Rheum*, 1992; 19:8, 1170-1172.

Hit and Run or Permanent Hit? Is There Evidence for a Microbial Cause of Rheumatoid Arthritis? GR Burmester, W Solbach, *J Rheum*, 1992; 18:10, 1443-1447.

Pathogenesis of Rheumatoid Arthritis, K Sewell, D Trentham, *Lancet*, Jan. 30, 1993; 341: 283-286.

Rheumatoid Arthritis: How Well Do the Theories Fit the Evidence? J McCulloch, PM Lydyard, GAW Rook, *Clin Exp Immuno*, 1993; 92:1-6.

A Reappraisal of the Evidence that Rheumatoid Arthritis and Several Other Idiopathic Diseases Are Slow Bacterial Infections, GAW Rook, PM Lydyard, JL Stanford, *Ann Rheum Dis*, 1993; 52: S30-8.

Is Rheumatoid Arthritis Caused by an Infection? RJR McKendry, *Lancet*, May 27, 1995; 345: 1319-20.

Antibiotic Therapy for Rheumatoid Arthritis, DE Trentham, RA Dynesius-Trentham, *Rheum Dis Clin N Am*, August 1995; 21:3: 817-834.

Mycoplasmas in Rheumatoid Arthritis and Other Human Arthritides, D Taylor-Robinson, T Schaeverbeke, *J Clin Pathol*, 1996; 49: 718-782.

Systematic Detection of Mycoplasmas by Culture and Polymerase Chain Reaction (PCR) Procedures in 209 Synovial Fluid Samples, T Schaeverbeke, J Renaudin, M Clerc, L LeQuen, JP Vernhes, B DeBarbeyrac, B Bannwarth, CH Bebear, and J Dehais, *Br J Rheum*, 1997; 36:3, 310-314.

JUVENILE RA

Juvenile Rheumatoid Arthritis Inflammatory Eye Disease, Parasitization of Ocular Leukocytes by Mollicute-like Organisms, E Wirostko, L Johnson, W Wirostko, *J Rheum*, 1989; 16:11 1446-1451.

Epidemiology of Juvenile Rheumatoid Arthritis in Manitoba, Canada, 1975-92; Cycles in Incidence (JRA & *M pneumoniae*), K Oen, M Fast, B Postl, *J Rheum*, 22 (4) 1995; 745-750.

SCLERODERMA

Acid-Fast Bacteria as a Possible Cause of Scleroderma, AR Cantwell, Jr., E Craggs, JW Wilson, F Swatek, *Dermatologica*, 1968 136: 141-150.

Acid-Fast Bacteria in Scleroderma and Morphea, AR Cantwell, Jr., DW Kelso, *Arch of Derm*, 1971; 104:7, 21-25.

Histologic Forms Resembling "Large Bodies" in Scleroderma and Pseudoscleroderma, AR Cantwell, Jr., *Am J Derm*, 1980; 2:3, 273-276.

Photopheresis for Scleroderma? No! JF Fries, JR Seibold, TA Medsger, Jr., *J Rheum*, 1992; 19:7, 1011-1013.

Outcome Measurement in Scleroderma Clinical Trials, JE Pope, N Bellamy, *Sem in Arth and Rheum*, August, 22-23, 1993; 23:1.

Minocycline in Early Diffuse Scleroderma: A Pilot Open 12-Month Study in 11 Patients, CH Le, A Morales, DE Trentham (to be published in early 1998).

LUPUS

Ureaplasma Urealyticum and *Mycoplasma Hominis* in Women with Systemic Lupus Erythematosus, KS Ginsburg, RB Kudsin, CW Walter, PH Schur, *Arth & Rheum*, 1992; 35:4, 429-433.

Histologic Observations of Coccoid Forms Suggestive of Cell Wall Deficient Bacteria in Cutaneous and Systemic Lupus Erythematosus, AR Cantwell, Jr., DW Kelso, JE Jones, *Int J Derm*, 1982; 21:9, 526-37.

Varied Acid-Fast Bacteria in a Decropsied Case of Systemic Lupus Erythematosus with Acute Myocardial Infarction, AR Cantwell, Jr., JK Cove, Cutis, *Department of Dermatology, Southern California Permanente Medical Group*, Los Angeles, June 1984.

Parvovirus Infection Mimicking Systemic Lupus Erythematosus, G Nesher, TG Osborn, TL Moore, *Sem in Arth & Rheum*, 1995; 24:5, 297-303.

Induction of Cross-Reactive Anti-dsDNA Antibodies in Preautoimmune NZW/NZB Mice by Immunization with Bacterial DNA, GS Gilkeson, AMM Pippen, DS Pisetsky, *J Clin Invest*, 1995; 95:3, 1398-1402.

MYCOPLASMAS & OTHER L FORMS

Cell Wall Deficient Forms, LH Mattman, CRC Press, Cleveland, 1974.

Unexpectedly High Frequency of Antibody to *Mycoplasma Pneumoniae* in Human Sera as Measured by Sensitive Technique, H Brunner, B Prescott, H Greenberg, WD James, R Horswood, RM Chanock, *J Infect Dis*, 1977; 135, 524.

Arthritis Associated with *Mycoplasma Pneumoniae* Infection, A Ponka, *Scand J Rhu,* 1979; 8:27, 27-32.

Mycoplasmal Arthritis in Man, D Taylor-Robinson, *Isr J Med Sci,* 1981; 17: 7, 616-621.

Arthritis caused by *Mycoplasma Salivarium* in Hypogamma-gobulinaemia, AKL So, PM Furr, D Taylor-Robinson, ABD Webster, *Br J Rheum,* Mar. 5, 1983; 286: 762-763.

Infectious Agents, Immunity and Rheumatic Diseases, BJ Schwarts, *Arth & Rheum,* 1990; 33: 4, 457-465.

The Potential Role of Mycoplasmas as Autoantigens and Immune Complexes in Chronic Vascular Pathogenesis, HW Clark, *Am J of Primatology,* 1991; 24: 235-243.

Peculiar Properties of Mycoplasmas: The Smallest Self-replicating Prokaryotes, S Razin, *FEMS Micro Letters,* 100, 1992, 423-432.

Serological Diagnosis of *Mycoplasma Pneumoniae* Infections: A Critical Review of Current Procedures, E Jacobs, *Clin Infect Dis,* 1993; 17 (Suppl 1): S79-82.

Experience with New Techniques for the Laboratory Detection of *Mycoplasma Pneumoniae* Infection: Adelaide, 1978-1992, B Marmion, J Williamson, DA Worswick, TW Kok, RH Harris, *Clin Infect Dis,* 1993; 17.

Serological Diagnosis of *Mycoplasma Pneumoniae* Infections: A Critical Review of Current Procedures, E Jacobs, *Clin Infect Dis,* 1993; 17 (Suppl) S79-82.

Mycoplasma Hominis Septic Arthritis: Two Case Reports and Review, LM Luttrell, SS Kanj, GR Corey, RE Lins, RJ Spinner, WJ Mallon, DJ Sexton, *Clin Infect Dis,* 1994; 19: 1067-1070.

Mycoplasmas and Ureaplasmas in Patients with Hypogamma-obulinaemia and Their Role in Arthritis: Micro-Biological Observations over Twenty Years, PM Furr, D Taylor-Robinson,

ADB Webster, *Annals of the Rheum Dis,* 1994; 53: 183-187

Mycoplasma Genitalium in the Joints of Two Patients, D Taylor-Robinson, CB Gilroy, S Horowitz, J Horowitz, *Euro J of Clin Rheum,* 1994; 13, 1066-1069.

Mycoplasmas and Arthritis: a Systematic Culture Study of Synovial Fluids, T Schaeverbeke, H Renaudin, MC Clerc, B deBarbeyrac, C Bebear, B Barnswarth, J Dehais, *Arth & Rheu,* 1994 (abstract 925), 37:S315.

Mechanisms of Autoimmune Disease Induction: The Role of the Immune Response to Microbial Pathogens, SM Behar, SA Porcelli, *Arth & Rheum,* 1995; 38:4, 458-476.

The Phagocytosis of Mycoplasmas, AJ Marshall, RJ Mills, L Richards, *J Med Microbiol,* 1995; vol 43, 239-250.

A Disease Related Rheumatoid Factor Autoantibody Is Not Tolerized in a Normal Mouse: Implications for the Origins of Autoantibodies in Autoimmune Disease, LG Hannum, D Ni, AM Haberman, MG Weigert, MJ Shlomchik, *J Exp Med,* 1996; 184: 1269-1278.

Infections Due to Species of Mycoplasma and Ureaplasma: An Update, D Taylor-Robinson, *Clin Infect Dis,* 1996; 23: 671-684.

Mycoplasma Fermentans in Joints of Patients with Rheumatoid Arthritis and Other Joint Disorders, T Schaeverbeke, CB Gilroy, C Bebear, J Dehais, D Taylor-Robinson, *Lancet,* May 18, 1996; 347: 1418.

Micoplasma Interactions with the Immune System: Implications for Disease Pathology. Immune System Responses to Antigens from These Organisms Could Play Key Roles in Diseases Such as Rheumatoid Arthritis and AIDS, BC Cole, *Mycoplasmology & Immunol Div of ASM,* 1996; 62:9, 471-475.

Mycoplasmas: Sophisticated, Reemerging, and Burdened by Their Notoriety, JB Baseman, JG Tully, *CDC's Emerging Infectious Diseases,* 1997; 3:1.

OSTEOARTHRITIS

Doxycycline Inhibits Type XI Colagenolytic Activity of Extracts from Human Osteoarthritic Cartilage and of Gelatinase, LP Yu, GN Smith, Jr., KA Hasty, KD Brandt, *J Rheu,* 1991; 18:10, 1450-1452.

Tetracyclines Suppress Matrix Metalloproteinase Activity in Adjuvant Arthritis and in Combination with Flurbiprofin, Ameliorate Bone Damage, RA Greenwald, SA Moak, NS Rammamurthy, LM Golub, *J Rheu,* 1992; 19:6, 928-938.

REITER'S SYNDROME

Poststreptococcal Reactive Arthritis, MH Arnold, A Tyndall, *Ann Rhu Dis,* 1989; 48: 686-88.

Double-Blind, Placebo-Controlled Study of Three Month Treatment with Lymecycline in Reactive Arthritis, with Special Reference to Chlamydia Arthritis, A Lauhio, M Leirisalo-Repo, J Lahdevirta, P Saikku, H Repo, *Arth & Rheum,* 1991; 34:1, 6-14.

Recurrent Arthritis in Reiter's Syndrome: A Function of Inapparent Chlamydial Infection of The Synovium? MU Rahman, HR Schumacher, AP Hudson, Sem in Arth & Rheum, 21:4, 1992, 259-266.

Ureaplasma Ureallyticum in Reiter's Syndrome, S Horowitz, J Horowitz, D Taylor-Robinson, S Hukenik, RN Apte, J Ben-David, B Thomas, C Gilroy, *J Rheum,* 1994; 21:9, 877-882.

Molecular Detection of Bacterial DNA in Venereal-Associated Arthritis, F Li, R Bulbul, HR Schumacher, T Kieber-Emmons, PE Callegari, JM Von Feldt, D Norden, B Freundlich, B Wang, V Imonitie, CP Chang, I Nachamkin, DB Weiner, WV Williams, *Arth & Rheum,* 1996; 39-6, 950-958.

Reactive or Septic Arthritis. Comment on the Article by Li et al, T. Schaeverbeke, C Bebear, B Bannwarth, J Dehais, *Arth & Rheum,* 1997; 40:3, 592-592.

MISCELLANEOUS

Second International Symposium on the Immunotherapy of the Rheumatic Diseases: Concepts and Overview, *Clin and Exper Rheum II,* 1993; (Suppl 8): S1-S3.

The End of the Self, S Richardson, *Discover,* April 1996, 80-87.

Tetracyclines, Chloramphenicol, Erythromycin, Clindamycin, and Metronidazole, JD Smilack, WR Wilson, FR Cockerill, III, *Mayo Clin Proc,* 1991; 66: 1270-1280.

Penetration and Bactericidal Activity of Cefixime in Synovial Fluid, E Somekj, L Heifetz, M Dan, F PPoch, H Hafei, A Tanai, *Antimicrob Agents and Chemo,* ASM, 40:5; 1996, 1198-1200.

Additional Articles by Thomas McPherson Brown, M.D.

Defective Serum Chemotactic Capacity in Rheumatoid Arthritis, WM Attia, MKH Ali, LMA Abu-ghazalah, AH Shams, HW Clark, TMcP Brown, *Ann of Allergy,* 1983, 50: 4, 266-270.

Medium-dependent Properties of Mycoplasmas, HW Clark, JS Bailey, TMcP Brown, *Diag Microbiol Infect Dis,* 1985, 3; 283-294.

Detection of Mycoplasmas in Immune Complexes (abstract), HW Clark, MR Coker-Vann, JS Bailey, TMcP Brown, *Int'l Congress of the Int'l Org for Mycoplasmology,* 1986.

In-vitro Effect of Alpha-Interferon on Lymphocytes of Normal and Autoimmune Patients, AM Attallah, AD Steinberg, HW Clark, TMcP Brown, A Metwali, TA Fleisher, *Int Arch Allergy Appl Immun,* 1986, 513.

Detection of mycoplasmal antigens in immune complexes from rheumatoid arthritis synovial fluids, HW Clark, MR Coker-Vann, JS Bailey, TMcP Brown, *Ann of Allergy,* 1988, 60: 5; 394-398.

How You Can Help

The Road Back Foundation was formed as a not-for-profit, 501(c)3 corporation in 1993 by grateful patients, their families, and supporters, to continue the pioneering work of Thomas McPherson Brown, M.D. The Foundation supports studies and clinical trials of antibiotics in connective tissue disease, and provides the latest comprehensive information on these diseases free of charge to patients and doctors around the world.

The Harvard Medical School study of minocycline in scleroderma, described in this book and subsequently reported in *The Lancet*, was sponsored primarily by The Road Back Foundation, and secondarily by the National Institutes of Health. Other present or pending Road Back Foundation–sponsored research projects include Juvenile Rheumatoid Arthritis, fibromyalgia, and a statistical analysis of minocycline in scleroderma based on a significantly larger patient sampling.

In addition, the Foundation maintains a popular, informative web site, publishes a newsletter to patients and physicians, sponsors physician conferences, and maintains a fast-growing network of patient support groups throughout the United States, Canada, and abroad.

The Road Back Foundation's only source of income is gifts and contributions. Its only expenditures are in support of laboratory and clinical research, and for education of patients and physicians.

Send your 100-percent tax deductible contribution to:

The Road Back Foundation
P.O. Box 447
Orleans, MA 02653

Write to ask about tax-deductible contribution for a Thomas McPherson Brown Research Endowment in Rheumatology, in explicit affiliation with Harvard Medical School.

For the address and phone number of the support group nearest to you write to the above address or visit the Road Back Foundataion's web site at www.roadback.org.